engender

tactical medic

p.13 economies + diseconomies of scale

<u>Public Health: What It Is and How It Works.</u>
  by Turnock
  Ch. 6 Medicare 74+, Title XVIII
        Medicaid p.82-8, Title XIX

Health Care Financing Review - journal
US Dpt of Commerce Statistical Abstract of the US.
★ Journal of Health Politics, Policy + Law
purchase $60/yr   p.76   p.105
                                           α trust
APHA journal $200/'95   VA state bar
                                                    assoc.
    p.28 more
          <u>Journals</u>   viol. Shum
      Applied Economics
      Journal of Health Economics   p.108 RLM
      Journal of Economics

                        p.20 sued
                             good rapport

The Health Care Marketplace

Springer
New York
Berlin
Heidelberg
Barcelona
Budapest
Hong Kong
London
Milan
Paris
Singapore
Tokyo

The Health Care Marketplace

Warren Greenberg, Ph.D.

Professor of Health Economics
Department of Health Services Management and Policy
School of Public Health and Health Services
The George Washington University
Washington, D.C.

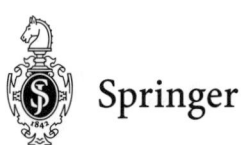 Springer

Warren Greenberg
The George Washington University
Department of Health Services Management and Policy
600 21st Street, N.W.
Washington, D.C. 20052
USA

Permission to reprint pages 99, 105, 108, 111, 113–116, 119–120, 122–129, 134–136, 144–148, and 159–161 of *Competition, Regulation, and Rationing in Health Care* has been granted. Used with permission from *Competition, Regulation, and Rationing in Health Care* by W. Greenberg (Chicago: Health Administration Press), 99–161.

Library of Congress Cataloging-in-Publication Data
Greenberg, Warren, 1943–
    The health care marketplace / Warren Greenberg.
      p. cm.
    ISBN 0-387-98457-7 (alk. paper)
    1. Medical economics—United States. I. Title.
RA410.53.6745 1998
338.4'33621'0973—dc21   97-47489

Printed on acid-free paper.

© 1998 Springer-Verlag New York, Inc.
All rights reserved. This work may not be translated or copied in whole or in part without the written permission of the publisher (Springer-Verlag New York, Inc., 175 Fifth Avenue, New York, NY 10010, USA), except for brief excerpts in connection with reviews or scholarly analysis. Use in connection with any form of information storage and retrieval, electronic adaptation, computer software, or by similar or dissimilar methodology now known or hereafter developed is forbidden.
The use of general descriptive names, trade names, trademarks, etc., in this publication, even if the former are not especially identified, is not to be taken as a sign that such names, as understood by the Trade Marks and Merchandise Marks Act, may accordingly be used freely by anyone.

Production managed by Bill Imbornoni; manufacturing supervised by Jeffrey Taub.
Typeset by Best-set Typesetter Ltd., Hong Kong.
Printed and bound by Edwards Brothers, Inc., Ann Arbor, MI.
Printed in the United States of America.

9 8 7 6 5 4 3 2 1

ISBN 0-387-98457-7 Springer-Verlag New York Berlin Heidelberg   SPIN 10663664

To Judith, Elyssa, and Shaked

Preface

This book is an economist's view of the health care marketplace. It examines the incentives of physicians, patients, firms and the role of government in the health care sector in a world of limited resources.

Several themes run through this book. First, health care is a business. To an economist this means that firms maximize profits. Perhaps this is not always so, but I have yet to see a better theory of how health care firms behave. The health care industry, therefore, is not much different in economic terms from other industries. At one time, economists pointed to the asymmetry of information between the physician provider and the patient as one difference between health care and other industries. Physicians often know a great deal about treating an illness while the patient knows little or nothing. But the movement toward managed care in the United States has partially closed the information gap (although perhaps creating other problems). Indeed, the advent of managed care has propelled health care into a business.

Information is another theme of the book. How can patients, physicians, and managed care plans grasp all the information they need on the complexities of health care? What is the most efficient way to provide information on the quality of a hospital or a physician? On what basis can managed care plans be evaluated? Is the purchase of a managed care plan any more or less complicated than the purchase of an automobile? Why aren't there greater incentives for managed care plans to advertise the quality of their plans?

Legal intervention in the health care industry is another thrust of the book. A representative legal case at the end of nine of the chapters illustrates how the health care market works in actual practice. Antitrust, a form of government intervention, has been an influence on the development of the health care marketplace. Judicial decisions on the purchase of health insurance in the workplace have affected employer-based health insurance. Malpractice and tort law have affected the cost and quality of health care.

I frequently borrow from the industrial organization (analysis of market structure, conduct, and performance) of other industries to illustrate the economics of the health care industry. People employed in the health care industry or studying health administration, health policy, or business programs may be surprised to find that the health care industry can be analyzed like other industries. I also borrow from the health care systems of Canada, Israel, and the Netherlands, in which the roles of the market and government in health care are quite different from each other and from those in the United States. The fact that the employer in these countries has virtually no role in the provision of health insurance might be a lesson for the United States.

The U.S. health care marketplace is in transition. Until the early 1980s, insuring organizations reimbursed physicians and hospitals with little regard to the cost of care. With the growth of cost-conscious managed care plans, physicians and hospitals have consolidated and merged.

Health care reform, in spite of the failure in 1994 of President Clinton's proposal, is still a necessity. It is not a concern if not everyone in a population has a video cassette recorder, but it is a concern if a large percentage of a population does not have health insurance. Moreover, the presence of health insurance creates inefficiencies in the marketplace which distorts the demand for and supply of health care services.

I would like to thank many of colleagues for their helpful comments and insights at various stages of the book. In particular, Ted Frech, Jack Hadley, Fred Hellinger, Jack Meyer, Amy Sparks, and Wynand van de Ven, each contributed to the book's worth. My George Washington University research assistants, Glen Bedell, Jennifer Peters, Namrata Sen, Michelle Wilson, and Nicole Zoia, brought energetic prowess to the project. Dr. Richard F. Southby, Chair of the Department of Health Services, Management, and Policy and Associate Dean of the School of Public Health and Health Services, graciously provided me with the assistants as well as technical support.

WARREN GREENBERG

Contents

Preface vii

1. Introduction to the Economics of Health Care 1
2. Physician Services Industry 12
3. Hospital Industry 27
4. Insurance, Managed Care, and System Integration 43
5. Employer and Employee as Purchasers of
   Health Care Services 63
6. Health Insurance in the Public Sector 73
7. Long-Term Care Industry 91
8. Antitrust in the Health Care Sector 103
9. Regulation and Competition in Health Care 119
10. Technology and Rationing in Health Care 135
11. Insights from Canada, Israel, and the Netherlands 152

Index 165

1
Introduction to the Economics of Health Care

The industrial organization of the health care industry has changed dramatically over the last decade, although the underlying economics of health care has remained the same. The industrial organization of health care is now dominated by the intervention of the health insuring organization or the managed care firm into the health care marketplace. The financing of health care services is increasingly performed by aggressive insuring organizations rather than by health insurers who passively pay the health care bill.

Size and Growth of the Health Care Sector

Table 1-1 shows health care expenditures by major industry component for selected years from 1960 to 1995. Between 1960 and 1995, total health care expenditures increased more than 37 times; they grew more than 300 percent between 1980 and 1995.

Table 1-2 shows total health care expenditures as well as health care expenditures as a percentage of the gross domestic product (GDP), or the total of all goods and services produced in the United States, for selected years. The table confirms that not only are health care expenditures increasing absolutely, they are also increasing faster than the remainder of the economy.

Increasing health care expenditures do not necessarily mean that there are inefficiencies or economic imperfections in the industry. For example, with higher real incomes, individuals may desire more health care, suggesting that health care behaves like a "normal" good in which greater income spurs greater consumption of the good. Rapid technological change in health care coupled with substantial insurance coverage may engender growth in expenditures. The reasons for rising health care costs are fully discussed in Chapter 10.

2   1. Introduction to the Economics of Health Care

TABLE 1-1. National health care expenditures by type of expenditure: Selected calendar years 1960–1995

Type of expenditure	Amount in billions of dollars					
	1960	1970	1980	1990	1994	1995
Total health care	23.6	63.8	217.0	614.7	827.9	878.8
Hospital care	9.3	28.0	102.7	256.4	335.0	350.1
Physician services	5.3	13.6	45.2	146.3	190.6	201.6
Dental services	2.0	4.7	13.3	31.6	42.1	45.8
Other professional services	0.6	1.4	6.4	34.7	49.1	52.6
Home health care	0.1	0.2	2.4	13.1	26.3	28.6
Drugs and other medical nondurables	4.2	8.8	21.6	59.9	77.7	83.4
Prescription drugs	2.7	5.5	12.0	37.7	51.3	55.5
Vision products and other medical durables	0.6	1.6	3.8	10.5	12.9	13.8
Nursing home care	0.8	4.2	17.6	50.9	72.4	77.9
Other personal health care	0.7	1.3	4.0	11.2	21.7	25.0

Source: Katharine R. Levit et al., "National Health Expenditures, 1995," *Health Care Financing Review*, 18 (Fall 1996): Table 1, p. 179.

TABLE 1-2. Gross domestic product (GDP) and total health care expenditures (HCE) as a percent of GDP: Selected calendar years 1960–1995

Year	GDP (billions of dollars)	HCE (billions of dollars)	HCE as percent of GDP
1960	527	26.9	5.1
1970	1,036	73.2	7.1
1980	2,784	247.2	8.9
1990	5,744	697.5	12.1
1992	6,244	834.2	13.4
1993	6,553	892.1	13.6
1994	6,936	937.1	13.5
1995	7,254	988.5	13.6

Source: Katharine R. Levit et al., "National Health Expenditures, 1995," *Health Care Financing Review*, 18 (Fall 1996): Table 8, p. 199.

Demand and Supply

Although the health care industry may have different characteristics than other industries, the principles of demand and supply are as applicable to health care as to other industries. Familiarity with these principles will improve one's understanding of how the health care industry behaves. The demand curve illustrated in Figure 1-1 slopes downward to the right. It shows the number of services that are demanded by patients or firms at a set of hypothetical prices. If the prices of health services are higher, fewer services are purchased than are purchased at lower prices. The supply curve illustrated in Figure 1-1 slopes upward to the right. It shows the number of services that a firm or medical professional provides at a set of hypothetical

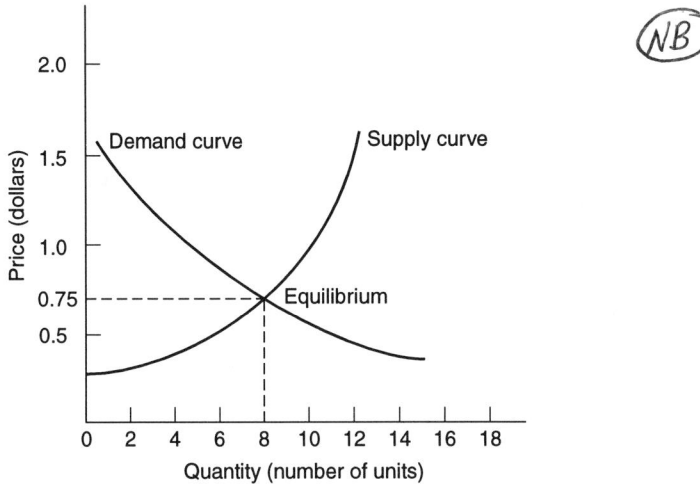

FIGURE 1-1. Supply and demand equilibrium

prices. The higher the price, the more services provided. If nursing personnel, for example, are paid overtime for working on the weekend, more nurses are willing to supply their services. In contrast, at low fees, fewer nurses have incentives to work.

The demand and supply curves for some health services deviate from the traditional downward and upward slopes. For example, the demand for life-saving insulin is not downward sloping for the diabetic but is closer to a vertical shape. This shape suggests that the amount of insulin demanded would be nearly the same regardless of the price charged.

The concepts of elasticity of demand and supply are used by economists to describe the shapes of the demand and supply curves. Elasticity of demand is defined as the relative change in quantity demanded of a good or service divided by the relative change in price. Since the relative change in quantity demanded of insulin is less than the relative change in price, the demand for insulin is relatively inelastic. If the relative change in quantity demanded is greater than the relative change in price, such as for many home care services, the demand is relatively elastic. Where relative changes in prices and quantity demanded are the same, the demand elasticity is termed unitary.

Elasticity of supply is defined as the relative change in quantity supplied divided by the relative change in price. For example, due in part to large capital requirements, new hospitals may not be built quickly in response to a relative increase in price. Supply of new hospitals may be regarded as relatively inelastic. In contrast, a relatively small increase in wages may induce a relatively large increase in unskilled home health care workers, making their supply curve relatively elastic.

4   1. Introduction to the Economics of Health Care

The intersection of demand and supply determines the equilibrium price of the good or service, as Figure 1-1 shows. The prices of goods and services may change, however, if the demand or the supply or both curves shift. For example, if more people become ill from an epidemic like AIDS, the demand curve will shift upward to the right for health services for AIDS patients. All things held equal, this shift will increase price, as shown in Figure 1-2. However, if there is an increase in supply of these health services, the supply curve will shift to the right. A new equilibrium price will be established that will depend on the relative shift of the demand and supply curves.

The demand curve for health services may also shift to the left, because, for example, individuals have lower incomes than previously; the supply of specialty physicians may shift to the left because of more severe licensing requirements. A new price is determined that depends on the relative shifts of the demand and supply curves.

Although the health care industry may have different attributes from those of other goods and services [Kenneth Arrow, "Uncertainty and the Welfare Economics of Medical Care," *American Economic Review*, 53 (1963): 941–973; Mark V. Pauly, "Is Medical Care Different?" in *Competition in the Health Care Sector: Past, Present, and Future*, ed. W. Greenberg (Germantown MD: Aspen Systems Corporation, 1978), pp. 11–35], the basic demand and supply curves of economics are still valuable in understanding the health care industry. For example, Arrow has suggested that the uncertainty of when illness may strike may make the health care industry different from other industries. Uncertainty, coupled with the potential high cost of illness, are the reasons for having health care insur-

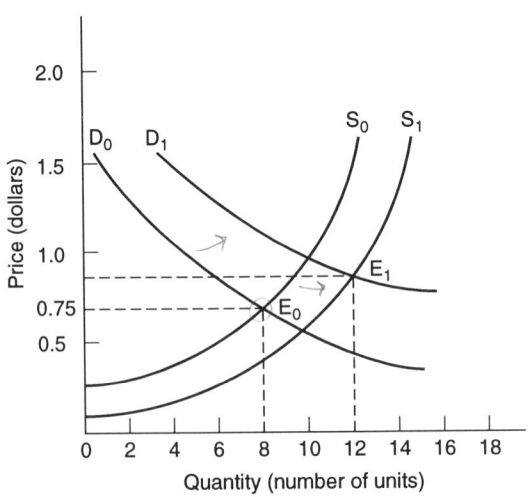

FIGURE 1-2. Shift in supply and demand curve

ance coverage. In addition, unlike other types of uncertain events such as a fire in one's home, health care insurance is subject to moral hazard. That is, when health care services are covered by insurance, more services are likely to be consumed than if consumers had to pay for the services themselves.

The presence of health insurance, however, can easily be integrated into the demand curve. An increase in traditional indemnity health insurance shifts a demand curve to the right. It also makes the demand curve more inelastic. Thus, as one would expect, the presence of insurance coverage can increase the prices and quantity of health care services. The presence of a managed care firm can shift the demand curve back down to the left (see Chapter 4).

According to Pauly, lack of information about the quality, nature, and price of health care services may make health care different from other industries. It may also affect the demand for health care. The demand curve for physician services, for example, can shift to the right if a physician suggests additional procedures about which the patient has little information and the patient follows the physician's recommendation. An asymmetry of information exists between a knowledgeable physician and an unknowledgeable patient. On the other hand, the patient on repeated visits for a chronic disease may know what to expect from the physician; sometimes, the physician knows little about the possible outcome.

Industrial Organization of Market Structures

Economists have observed that the number and size distribution of firms vary among industries. Variation may occur because of differences in barriers to entry to the industry. Barriers to entry measure how difficult it is for firms to enter an industry. For example, barriers to entry in the form of special licensing requirements prevent many highly educated persons from becoming physicians. Hospitals may find it difficult to enter geographical regions because of state certificate-of-need laws that require hospitals to demonstrate a need for their services before entering a market. By categorizing the size, distribution, and barriers to entry of firms in any industry, a beginning can be made in predicting profits, innovation, quality of service, and other elements of performance.

Pure Competition Model

The pure competition model (Figure 1-3) is used by economists to describe an efficient structure of an industry. It is efficient because the incremental cost of producing another unit of the service is equal to the average cost of producing the service as well as the price of the service. A competitive rate of return is necessary to keep firms from leaving the industry. The pure competition model is also characterized by a large number of competing firms and no barriers to entry for firms that seek to enter. The output of the

1. Introduction to the Economics of Health Care

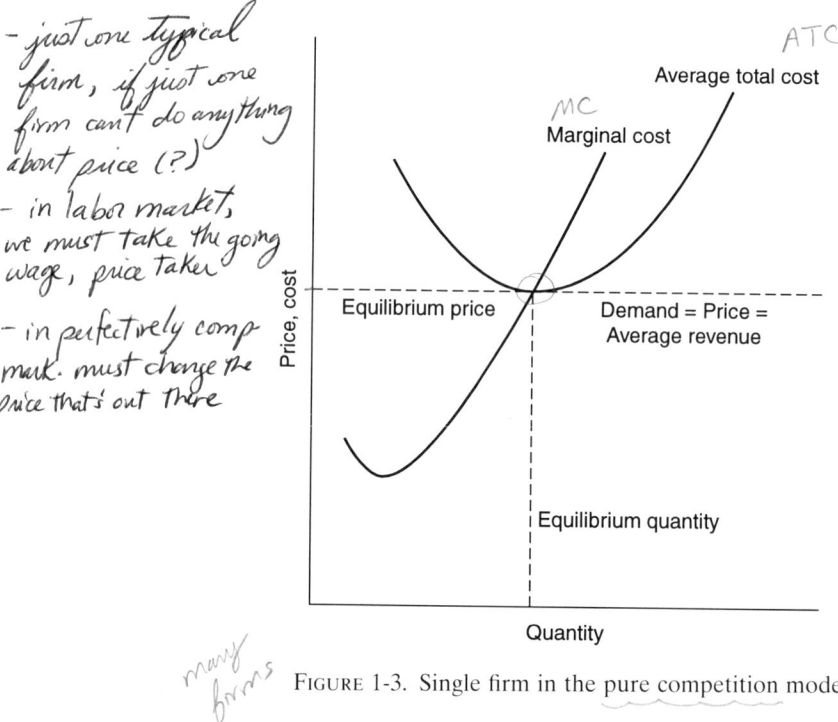

FIGURE 1-3. Single firm in the pure competition model

firms is a homogeneous good or service; no buyer would have a preference of one seller over another. Consumers have complete information about prices and quality of goods or services. No single seller under pure competition can raise its price without another seller potentially undercutting it with a lower price. Therefore, each firm in pure competition faces a perfectly elastic or horizontal demand curve.

Rarely can an industry in the economy be described as perfectly competitive. Even farmers who produce the same type of corn are located in different geographic areas, necessitating different costs and prices. Nevertheless, economists use the pure competition model as a polar example of an efficient industry. Figure 1-3, above, shows a single firm in the pure competition model.

Monopoly Model

The monopoly model (Figure 1-4) depicts a structure in which an industry consists of a single firm rather than a large number of firms. The single firm is the industry. High barriers to entry make it impossible for potential new entrants to erode any monopoly profits. The monopoly firm is not efficient since the prices charged are in excess of the marginal cost of producing the service.

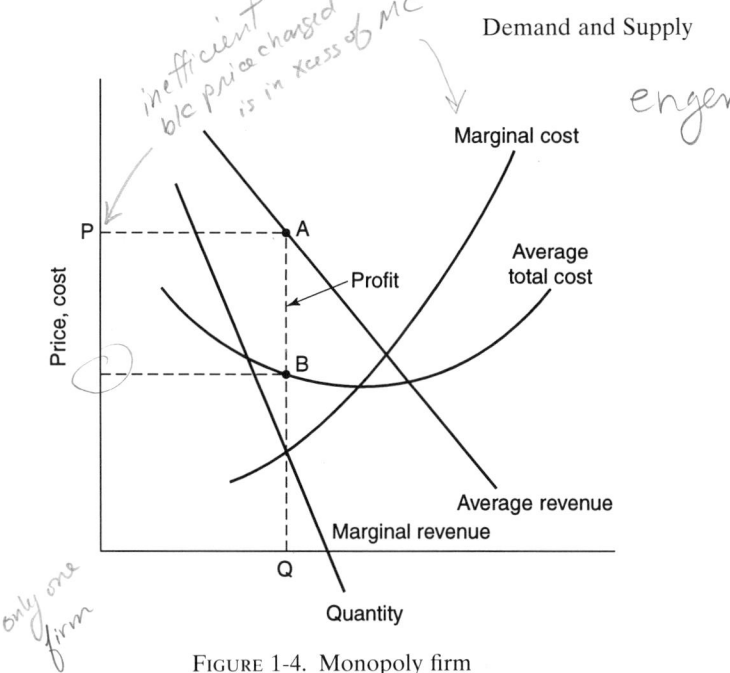

FIGURE 1-4. Monopoly firm

Monopolists charge prices that maximize their profits. If too high a price is charged, less of the good or service is sold. If too low a price is charged, total revenues are reduced. To maximize profits, monopolists charge a price and produce an output on the demand curve that is directly above the intersection of the marginal cost and marginal revenue curves.

It is uncommon to find a monopolist for a long period in the health care sector or in any other industry because high profits generally engender entry. However, patents on new products such as pharmaceuticals create barriers to entry for new competitors enabling the existing firm to achieve a monopoly structure and monopoly profits.

A monopoly has the ability to charge multiple prices for a single service. By charging a number of different prices to the same consumer or to different consumers for the same service (price discrimination), a monopolist can earn even greater profits. For example, Reuben A. Kessel ["Price Discrimination in Medicine," *Journal of Law and Economics*, 1 (1958): 20–53] examined physician pricing in the early 1900s and mid-1950s. Kessel found that physicians charged different prices to different patients depending on the elasticity of demand. Patients with higher incomes and a lower elasticity of demand were charged higher prices. Patients with lower incomes and greater elasticity of demand were charged lower prices. In this way physicians were able to increase their revenue (and profits) while at the same time making health care more accessible to a greater number of patients.

Monopolistic Competition and Oligopoly Models

Since the pure competition market structure is primarily used as a model and monopoly is rare, economists put most industries into monopolistically competitive or oligopolistic categories. A monopolistically competitive industry is one in which a number of firms compete but each firm has some ability to raise its price without all of its sales being taken away by its rivals. The ability of a firm to raise its price may be based on how a firm is able to differentiate itself from its competitors. For example, although one physician group may compete with another, it may differentiate itself based on convenience, perceived quality, or fee schedule.

Many industries are monopolistically competitive. The beer, restaurant, and management consulting industries, each consist of a number of firms competing with a slightly differentiated product for the consumer's business. In the health care industry, nursing homes in a large metropolitan area compete on reputation, perceived quality, price, and convenience. Third-party insuring organizations and managed care plans attempt to differentiate themselves by price, terms of coverage, convenience in filing claims, accessibility, or quality of physicians in their benefits plan.

In oligopolistic industries, instead of a large number of competitors, only a few firms compete on price, quality, convenience, or other dimensions. There may be only two firms, termed a duopoly, or as many as eight firms. With only a few firms in an industry, each firm must pay attention to how the other firms compete. For example, if firm A lowers its price, firm B must also be prepared to lower its price or compete on a nonprice basis. Indeed, Firm A and its rivals may pursue an infinite number of competitive strategies. One such strategy is collusion. Firm A may attempt to collude with Firm B on price, on division of markets, or on any other basis.

Firms may maximize profits as a group if they collude. This is a concern of most economists when a few firms dominate the market. However, collusion is not easily accomplished. Each firm has an incentive to break away from a collusive group since it can make greater profits when it acts independently. Firms may find ways to break away from the group without ready detection from other firms in the industry. For example, in the retail automobile industry, the actual prices of transactions between the seller and consumers can vary in the privacy of the dealership when other sellers are not present to check the retail selling price. Moreover, if a few firms in the market collude and set prices at the monopoly level, they must take into consideration the possibility of potential entry of a new competitive firm.

Depending on barriers to entry and the propensity for collusion, industries with oligopolistic market structures may realize supranormal profits. Prices may be above or at marginal cost curves. If prices are above marginal cost, inefficiency results. Additional factors must also be taken into consideration in evaluating performance. To what extent, for example, is there innovation in the industry? Are profits short-run, and will they not be sustained over the long run? Does government intervention account for higher profits?

The physician services industry (Chapter 2), hospital industry (Chapter 3), insuring organization and managed care industries (Chapter 4), and long-term care industry (Chapter 7) fall into the monopolistic competitive or oligopolistic market structures. The cited chapters ascertain performance in these industries.

Public Goods

Public goods are goods or services from whose benefits individuals cannot be excluded. The defense of the nation is often cited as an example of a public good since no one can be excluded from its potential benefits. No firms in the private marketplace "produce" defense since one need not pay to receive the "benefits." The defense of the nation is produced only by the government, which may elect to contract with private suppliers to build airplanes, missiles, and other military hardware.

There are few public goods in the economy and fewer still in the health care industry. Basic biomedical research from which benefits may accrue to an entire nation may be an example of a public good in health care. In contrast, the results of applied private medical research by pharmaceutical firms may be sold in the private marketplace as new drugs.

Externalities

Externalities are goods and services for which the benefits and costs accrue not only to the buyer of the service but to others as well. Thus, an individual who pays for a vaccination not only may not contract a disease but also may prevent others from contracting the disease. Thus, vaccinations may be termed a positive externality, or social benefit. If the social benefit exceeds the benefit to the individual consumer, society as a whole may want to subsidize the provision of vaccines.

Negative externalities, or social costs, occur when others beside the buyer incur the costs of the good or service. Individuals who do not smoke experience a negative externality when they bear the health risk of secondhand smoke. An efficient government response may be to tax cigarettes in order to reduce consumption and the size of the negative externality.

Distribution of Health Care Services

Economists are concerned mostly with efficiency. There is no economic theory of what constitutes an equitable distribution of health care insurance or health care services; efficiency simply dictates that individuals optimally purchase health care services as long as the benefits received (however measured) exceed the costs. Yet, because health services can be of value in the preservation of life or the quality of life, the nature of the distribution of health care services throughout the entire population, the number of individuals who are uninsured, and the quality of services individuals receive are of societal and political concern.

Process of Creative Destruction

Industries are not static; they are constantly changing. Economist Joseph Schumpeter envisioned a "process of creative destruction" [*Capitalism, Socialism and Democracy* (New York: Harper and Row, 1942), pp. 81–86], in which competition within existing industries is overtaken by new industries that render the older industries obsolete. A recent example is the replacement of the typewriter industry by the computer industry. Even within the computer industry, the main frame computer has been replaced, in large part, by the personal computer. The record and tape industries have been overtaken by compact discs.

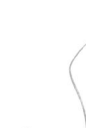

The health care industry is no exception to the process of creative destruction. Rising health care costs in fee-for-service medicine have encouraged health maintenance organizations (HMOs), preferred provider organizations (PPOs), and other forms of managed care to enter the health care financing marketplace. Rising in-patient hospital costs have encouraged a shift to out-patient settings. Rising physician specialist fees have encouraged delivery systems to favor the use of primary care physicians. In the 1970s, for example, the growth of HMOs increased most rapidly in states where health care costs in a mostly fee-for-service environment had grown fastest [Lawrence G. Goldberg and Warren Greenberg, "The Determinants of HMO Enrollment and Growth," *Health Services Research*, 16 (Winter 1981): 421–438].

Managed Care and the Health Care Marketplace

The advent of managed care has contributed substantially in making the health care industry a health care marketplace. The concept of managed care pervades each chapter in this book. Although managed care is discussed fully in Chapter 4, an understanding of the basic concept of managed care will be helpful now.

Managed care is the transformation of the passive health insurer, which simply paid the providers for whatever services were rendered, to the cost-conscious insuring organization that actively attempts to control costs and affect quality in the health care marketplace. It may selectively contract with a group of physicians or hospitals based on price and perceived quality.

It may deny in-hospital admission for some ailments and curtail length of stay. It may recommend more cost-effective means of treatment.

The managed care firm impedes on physician autonomy. But if the physician can still be called the captain of the health care team, the managed care firm is the first mate [Victor R. Fuchs, *Who Shall Live?* (New York: Basic Books, 1974), Chapter 3].

2
Physician Services Industry

Although physician services account for less than 20 percent of the expenditures in the health care industry, physicians order tests, procedures, hospital stays, and medical examinations equal to approximately 70 percent of the expenditures in the industry. The physician services industry can be viewed primarily as monopolistically competitive with many oligopolistic elements in local communities. The physician services industry has had and continues to have some monopolistic characteristics, such as high entry barriers for allied health practitioners who might compete with physicians as well as licensing requirements for new physicians. Physicians, however, may compete for contracts with managed care plans or compete in a fee-for-service environment.

Structure of the Physician Services Market

In 1994, 684,414 physicians were involved in patient care in the United States, an increase of 106.9 percent from the 330,824 physicians in 1970 [American Medical Association, *Physician Characteristics and Distribution in the U.S.*, 1995/96 edition, p. 23]. At the same time, the U.S. population grew only 28.1 percent, although the number of individuals over age 65 grew by 66 percent [U.S. Department of Commerce, Department of Data Survey and Planning, "Table 14. Resident Population by Age and Sex: 1970 to 1995," *Statistical Abstract of the United States, 1996*, p. 15].

The number of female physicians grew nearly threefold, from 35,636 in 1970 to 104,194 in 1994 ["Physician Characteristics and Distribution in the U.S.," p. 10]. Female physicians, however, tend to work fewer hours than male physicians [Robert H. Lee and Thomas A. Mroz, "Family Structure and Physicians' Hours in Large, Multispecialty Groups," *Inquiry*, 28 (Winter 1991): 366–374, p. 366]. Thus, examining the statistic "number of physicians" alone is not sufficient to evaluate fully the potential supply of physicians or the strength of the demand pressures on any one physician or physicians as a group. Moreover, phrases such as physician "glut" or physician "surplus" have little economic meaning. A glut or surplus means that prices or fees should decline to the competitive equilibrium level at which a greater number of services will be performed. In a normally functioning marketplace, a glut or surplus should mean good news for consumers and bad news for the sellers of the service as prices fall and quantity of services increase.

Physicians have also been increasingly practicing in a group setting. In 1996, one-third of all physicians practiced in a group with more than 100 physicians [American Medical Association, *Medical Groups in the U.S., A Survey of Practice Characteristics*, 1996 edition, Table 3-1, p. 7]. One reason for a greater number of groups may be economies of scale of group practice. According to a survey of the empirical evidence on economies of scale, Gregory C. Pope and Russel T. Burge found that physicians who practice in groups realize greater productivity than those who practice solo, although diseconomies of scale begin to appear in larger groups ["Inefficiencies in Physician Practices," *Advances in Health Economics and Health Services Research*, 13 (1992): 129–164]. Another advantage to group practice might be increased bargaining power in negotiations with managed care plans or a desire to participate and provide services to HMOs. In a survey conducted by the American Medical Association, a large percentage of physicians had contracted with managed care plans in 1994. Approximately 72 percent of physicians had contracted with an HMO; approximately 42 percent had contracted with an individual practice association (IPA), where physicians who practice in their offices receive a reduced fee or capitated amount for the patients they see; approximately 85 percent had contracted with a preferred provider organization (PPO) where physicians accept reduced fees and utilization review in return for a greater number of patients [American Medical Association, *Physician Marketplace Statistics*, November 1994, p. 129].

Physicians have also aligned themselves with hospitals in vertically integrated networks or physician-hospital organizations (PHOs). Vertical integration is the combination of supplier and buyer organizations into a single firm. If U.S. Steel were to purchase General Motors Corporation, for example, the combination of steel and automobile companies would make it a vertically integrated firm. Economists have identified a number of potential benefits of vertical integration [Oliver E. Williamson, "Transaction-Cost Economics: The Governance of Contractual Relations," *Journal of Law and Economics*, 22 (1979): 233–261; Kathryn M. Fenton and Barry C. Harris, "Vertical Integration and Antitrust in Health Care Markets," *Antitrust Bulletin*, 39 (Summer 1994): 421–438]. Some benefits to physicians might be a reduction in transactions costs, or the costs of negotiating with hospitals about referral patterns or terms of reimbursement, an increase in access to capital, and potential collaboration in negotiating with managed care plans. There is no accurate count of the number of PHOs. A 1994 survey found that 75 percent of PHOs were less than 25 months old and involved more specialists than primary care physicians [Ernst & Young LLP, *Physician-Hospital Organizations Profile 1995*, February 1995, pp. 1, 2].

Information Asymmetries

When a pair of shoes is purchased, the buyer may know nearly as much about the product as does the seller. The buyer can try on the shoes or even return them if they are not up to the buyer's expectations. The buyer can ask questions of the salesperson about the quality of the shoes or rely on advertising by the retailer or manufacturer.

In contrast, individuals visit physicians precisely because they do not know what ails them. Physicians may know a great deal or less about a particular illness, but in general, they know more than the patient. Sometimes physician visits are for chronically recurring illnesses, in which case the patient may be cognizant about the course of treatment.

This asymmetry of information may provide an incentive for the physician to perform a greater number of services than would be the case without asymmetry of information: the physician can make additional income from services of which the patient does not know the necessity. This would especially be true if the patient were insured, in which case the out-of-pocket costs to the patient are reduced. Supplier-induced demand is when physicians increase demand beyond that which would be the case in a market without asymmetries.

Supplier-Induced Demand

Supplier-induced demand is difficult to ascertain and even more difficult to measure. Suppose, for example, a McDonald's restaurant has just opened in a neighborhood. If individuals patronize this restaurant, it might simply mean that the travel cost of visiting this new McDonald's is less than the cost of visiting another McDonald's instead of demand being created. A decrease in travel costs means a decline in the overall price (the sum of pecuniary and travel costs), which suggests that the quantity demanded would increase regardless of demand creation. Similarly, an increase in number of physicians in an area means reduced travel costs and therefore a greater "demand" for physician services.

Before the substantial growth of managed care in the early 1990s, a number of studies showed positive relationships between number of physicians and higher prices and increased utilization, precisely the result that economic theory would not predict. For example, Cromwell and Mitchell found that surgeons' fees and utilization are higher in areas where there is a greater number of surgeons [Jerry Cromwell and Janet B. Mitchell, "Physician-Induced Demand for Surgery," *Journal of Health Economics*, 5 (1986): 296–313]. Waiting time and travel costs are essentially held constant here because they are far less significant in receiving surgery than in receiving primary care.

Some economists suggest that attempts to examine the extent of supplier-induced demand should ascertain any "positive increment in health status" that may have resulted from an increase in demand for physician services [Roberta Labelle, Greg Stoddart, and Thomas Rice, "A Re-examination of the Meaning and Importance of Supplier-Induced Demand," *Journal of Health Economics*, 13 (1994): 347–368]. If health status improved, the increased number of services stemmed from patients who simply needed more services; if health status showed no improvement, supplier-induced demand may have existed. Mark V. Pauly ["Editorial: A Re-examination of the Meaning and Importance of Supplier-Induced Demand," *Journal of Health Economics*, 13 (1994): 369–372], however, rejects the use of health status as a measure to explain supplier-induced demand because other reasons, including reassurance and freedom from anxiety, may induce individuals to see physicians. Moreover, Pauly suggests that even if health status were to improve, it would say nothing about the creation of demand because improved health may not have been worth its cost.

Purported increases in demand may also be exaggerated because of the presence of insurance. If there are increases in the demand for physician services when these services are covered by insurance, it may mean that the cause of the increased demand is simply reduced patient out-of-pocket cost.

Physician as Agent for the Patient

Demand inducement that leads to no benefits to the patient from the physician's service would violate the physician's position as agent for the patient. As agent for the patient, the physician as an informed provider of services has an obligation to recommend office visits, tests and procedures, hospitals, and hospital utilization that would be in the best interest of the patient.

But although in theory the physician is the agent for the patient, physicians have not necessarily acted on behalf of the patient. Jean M. Mitchell and Elton Scott report, for example, that physicians who own their own physical therapy and rehabilitation facilities refer patients to these units at a greater rate than physicians who do not own such facilities ["Physician Ownership of Physical Therapy Services," *Journal of the American Medical Association*, 268 (1992): 2055–2059]. Mitchell and Scott found that charges per patient and profits were also higher in these joint venture facilities.

In addition, diagnostic imaging services and charges for the Medicare population were greater for services performed in a physician's office compared to services performed by off-site radiologists [Bruce J. Hillman et al., "Physicians' Utilization and Charges for Outpatient Diagnostic Imaging in a Medicare Population," *Journal of the American Medical Association*, 268 (1992): 2050–2054].

A response to the convenience needs of the patient may explain greater use of services in a physician's office. Nevertheless, these studies raise questions about whether the physician is an agent for the patient. And there are some egregious examples that are in no doubt. For example, National Medical Enterprises pleaded guilty in 1994 of paying kickbacks for referrals to its large chain of psychiatric hospitals ["Hospital Chain Sets Guilty Plea," *New York Times*, June 29, 1994, p. D1]. General medical hospitals also appear to have paid physicians (fee splitting) for referrals ["Hospitals That Need Patients Pay Bounties for Doctors' Referrals," *Wall Street Journal*, February 27, 1989, p. 1.]

The issue of the physician as agent for the patient may also appear in quality of care concerns. A recent study found that physicians do no better than patients themselves in choosing high-volume hospitals (a proxy measure for quality) for cardiac surgery for their patients [Lawrence G. Goldberg and Warren Greenberg, "Are Physicians Agents for Their Patients? The Choice of Hospital for Cardiac Surgery," unpublished manuscript, 1997].

How Should Physicians Be Paid?

Most goods and services command a price or fee based on supply and demand. Because of the presence of insurance, which may distort demand, and the asymmetry of information for physician services, physicians have generally been paid in ways that may be only loosely related to supply and demand.

Many fee-for-service insurers have paid physicians on a usual, customary, and reasonable (UCR) basis. Under this system, physicians are paid the lowest of their usual charges for a procedure or at the percentile (usually 70 to 90 percent) of fees paid to other physicians in the same specialty in the same geographic area (the customary fee). This lower fee is termed the reasonable fee. However, under UCR, physicians have little incentive to keep fees low since a higher fee means, at worst, that the physician receives the UCR fee. Indeed, the insurer then adds the higher fee to the customary component calculation of the UCR for other physicians.

Under the Medicaid program (Chapter 6), many states pay physicians a flat fee for particular procedures, often below the fee dictated by supply and demand and below the fee paid by the private sector and Medicare. In 1993, Medicaid fees were approximately 47 percent of the fees the private sector paid physicians [Physician Payment Review Commission (PPRC), *1994*

Annual Report to Congress, p. 352]. New York state, for example, pay only $11.00 for a new patient office visit [PPRC, *1994 Annual Report to Congress*, Table 18-4, p. 356]. In addition, Medicaid fees for physicians are only approximately 73 percent of what Medicare pays [PPRC, *1994 Annual Report to Congress*, p. 352]. This low flat fee results in fewer physician services supplied than would be the case under competitive supply and demand conditions. In addition, in response to lower fees, physicians may unbundle procedures, ask patients to return more often for return visits, charge for telephone calls, or reduce the length of time for each visit.

Under the Medicare program (Chapter 6), physicians have been paid under a resource-based relative value scale (RBRVS) since 1992, replacing a traditional UCR payment mechanism. Under RBRVS, a physician is paid Medicare-determined costs of practice regardless of the demand for the services for more than 7,000 services, visits, and procedures. The costs include physician and nonphysician input, the costs of malpractice premiums, and adjustments for geographic location, multiplied by the total work effort of the physician for the procedure, including time, mental effort, technical skill, and stress in performing the procedures [James R. Baumgardner, "Medicare Physician-Payment Reform and the Resource-Based Relative Value Scale: A Re-creation of Efficient Market Prices," *American Economic Review*, September 1992, pp. 1027–1030].

Under the RBRVS system, physicians of differing quality each receive the same rate. Factors such as the skill and personal manner of the physician, which may influence demand, are not captured by this rate. The difficulties in the calculation of a "relative value scale"—the relative value for each medical service compared to all the other medical services for conversion into dollars—as well as the calculation of the update of the relative value scale on a yearly basis suggest that the RBRVS system does not arrive at fees resembling those realized in competitive markets.

The RBRVS system was not intended to control physician fees or expenditures but simply to alter the distribution of fees paid to various physician specialties. It was believed that UCR had resulted in a system in which physicians in the surgical specialties and the diagnostic testing that were nearly completely covered by insurance had much greater incomes than family practitioners and primary care physicians, where there was less insurance coverage. For example, in 1995, opthalmologists and anesthesiologists had earned average gross incomes of $194,000 and $203,000, respectively, while family practice physicians earned $124,000 [Physician Payment Review Commission, *1997 Annual Report to Congress*, Washington, DC, Table 16-1, p. 348].

The Medicare volume performance standards (MVPS) were instituted specifically to control physician costs. The MVPS measures the changes in physician practice costs and earnings over time. These changes are then compared to the target of the U.S. Congress of the annual rate of growth for physician expenditures [Jesse M. Levy et al., "Understanding the Medicare Fee Schedule and its Impact on Physicians Under the Final Rule," *Medical Care*, 30 (1992): Supplement, pp. NS80–NS93, NS85]. The differences between the actual and desired rate of physician expenditure growth are reflected in a new conversion factor update [Levy et al., NS85, NS86]. Thus, under the MVPS, physicians who practice a less invasive and less costly medicine will receive the same conversion update as physicians who practice a more costly medicine, leaving no incentive to practice in a cost-conscious manner.

The RBRVS system also exerted regulatory pressure on the limits of balance billing, or the amount that physicians could charge above Medicare's fee schedule [Levy et al., NS80]. These limits were first set in 1993 to be no more than 9.25% above the fee schedule regardless of the quality of the physician or the demand for his or her services [Levy et al., NS80].

The RBRVS is theoretically a model of a perfectly competitive economic system under which the fees a physician receives are equal to the marginal cost of providing the service [Edmund R. Becker et al., "Refinement and Expansion of the Harvard Resource-Based Relative Value Scale: The Second Phase," *American Journal of Public Health*, 80 (1990): 799–803]. Each physician, however, has a different marginal cost curve as well as a different patient mix and a different demand curve. Thus, even if marginal costs and demand could be perfectly measured, there would still be imperfections surrounding each physician's demand and supply curve. Moreover, the incentives to physicians to control costs are quite weak.

The RBRVS system is a system of fees paid by the government (the buyer) for each of the covered physician procedures. Unlike the typical marketplace transaction, the seller does not set the fees nor is there any negotiation between buyer and seller. As managed care plans grow, there seems to be a shift away from this means of reimbursement. When physicians are paid under managed care plans such as health maintenance organizations, they are paid on the basis of supply and demand for their services. Thus, a presumed shortage of primary care physicians will result in higher fees paid, and a presumed surplus of specialty care physicians will result in lower fees.

The average net income for family practice and primary care physicians for 1995 was $124,000, a 14.8 percent increase from 1992. All specialists made an average net income of $160,000 in 1995, a 2.5 percent decrease from 1992 [Physician Payment Review Commission, *1997 Annual Report to Congress*, Table 16-1, p. 348]. It is not surprising that salaries have declined for specialists and increased for family practice physicians since there has been such a large increase in managed care plans, which make relatively greater use of primary care physicians. Moreover, the RBRVS system has increased compensation to primary care physicians relative to specialty care physicians.

Do Physicians Respond to Market Incentives?

Under fee-for-service medicine, physicians have incentives to perform as many tests and procedures as they believe are required for patient care since, if the patient is insured, they will be reimbursed by the insuring organization. Under managed care, physicians can be at financial risk for procedures, tests, or the treatment of individual patients. One study has shown, for example, that a lower rate of hospitalization is associated with capitation payments to primary care physicians than with fee-for-service reimbursement [Alan L. Hillman, Mark V. Pauly, and Joseph J. Kerstein, "How Do Financial Incentives Affect Physicians' Clinical Decisions and the Financial Performance of Health Maintenance Organizations?" *New England Journal of Medicine*, 321 (1989): 86–92]. An even lower rate of hospitalization was found with salary-based payments, which sometimes involve peer review [Hillman, Pauly, and Kerstein, p. 89].

In his review of the impact of financial incentives on the behavior of physicians, Fred J. Hellinger found that incentives are key in the lower utilization rates enjoyed by managed care firms ["The Impact of Financial Incentives on Physician Behavior in Managed Care Plans: A Review of the Evidence," *Medical Care Research and Review*, 53 (1996): 294–314]. Hellinger also reviews studies that hold constant the disease that was treated (to control for case mix) as well as those that follow the same physician reimbursed on a fee-for-service or prepaid (managed care) basis (to control for physician practice preferences). In both the "same-disease" and "same-physician" studies it was shown that lesser utilization of health care services was found in managed care plans.

How Do Physicians Compete?

Competition among physicians takes place locally among primary care physicians and on a wider geographic scale among specialists: individuals might travel a greater distance to see a certain specialist. Competition also takes place between physicians (such as opthamologists and psychiatrists) and allied health practitioners (such as optometrists and psychologists). Physicians practicing in a fee-for-service environment also compete with physicians in managed care plans.

Physicians compete as would any other group of firms in a monopolistically competitive industry. Price competition occurs in the absence of insurance or the presence of a high deductible or copayment. Competition also takes place in professional demeanor, location, and waiting time. Physicians who are board-certified may emphasize the purported quality of their practice. Physicians may also compete to be preferred providers of managed care plans. Competition takes the form here of reduced fees, perceived quality of care, and prior practice of less intrusive medicine.

The quality of physician services has not been directly measured. The National Practitioner Data Bank, established in 1990, includes information such as malpractice suits brought against physicians who have had medical licenses or hospital privileges suspended for thirty days or more. The data bank, by law, is available only to hospitals; data in the data bank are specifically prohibited from distribution to the general public. Thus, hospitals serve as the clearinghouse for information on physicians ["Oversight, Phase 1: Keeping Records of Doctors With Records," *New York Times*, September 9, 1990, p. 26]. Hospitals can be held responsible if they have hired physicians who have adverse records in the bank. However, the release of this information to the public would have the important externality of informing individuals that not all physicians are of equal quality.

Physicians and Malpractice

Physicians are subject to malpractice litigation, although it is not clear that this is always due to poor performance. According to the liability laws under malpractice (the tort system), physicians are sued for negligent as well as nonnegligent incidents [Peter D. Jacobson, "Medical Malpractice and the Tort System," *Journal of the American Medical Association*, 262 (1989): 3320–3327]. Thus, it is not surprising that obstetricians and surgeons who have high-risk practices and more clearly determined outcomes are sued much more frequently than other kinds of physicians [Jacobson, p. 3321]. Most studies have concluded that physicians are most often sued when they do not have good rapport with the patient. Sloan has concluded that superior physicians have been sued on an equal basis with below-average physicians [Frank A. Sloan et al., "Medical Malpractice Experience of Physicians," *Journal of the American Medical Association*, 262 (1989): 3291–3297].

In 1987, six claims per one hundred physicians were filed [Jacobson, p. 3321], although most of the claims were settled without trial or won by the defendant [Jacobson, pp. 3321, 3322]. Studies have shown, however, that negligence is not insignificant [H. H. Hiatt, B. A. Barnes, T. A. Brennan et al., "Special Report: A Study of Medical Injury and Medical Malpractice," *New England Journal of Medicine*, 321 (1989): 480–484].

In order to curtail the current haphazard system of medical malpractice, Paul C. Weller, Joseph P. Newhouse, and Howard H. Hiatt propose a standard of strict liability that would end the accountability of individual physicians, and make the entire hospital responsible if malpractice were to be found ["Proposal for Medical Liability Reform," *Journal of the American Medical Association*, 267 (1992): 2355–2358]. The introduction of medical practice guidelines may also help reduce the uncertainty surrounding malpractice suits. Guidelines on the practice of medicine have been encouraged by the U.S. Congress and are currently being developed by professional medical societies [Deborah W. Garnick et al., "Can Practice Guidelines Reduce the Number and Costs of Malpractice Claims?" *Journal of the American Medical Association*, 266 (1991): 2856–2860]. Garnick et al. suggest that guidelines may improve quality of care, reduce the need for defensive medicine, and reduce administrative costs by focusing on national compared to community standards. Garnick et al. still caution, however, that large savings in malpractice costs probably will not be forthcoming from the use of these guidelines [p. 2859].

Health Care Marketplace

The American Medical Association was formed in 1847 by physicians who were concerned about their low incomes. One of its initial tasks was to reduce the number of medical schools and the number of physicians who could apply to medical school, shifting the supply curve of physicians to the left. However, it was believed that the "learned professions," including medicine, were exempt from antitrust action, and the AMA's activities to reduce the number of physicians were not challenged. When the learned profession exemption was taken away by the Supreme Court in 1975, it left the path open for Federal Trade Commission actions against the medical profession. The case brought by the Federal Trade Commission and eventually decided by the U.S. Supreme Court is reviewed in the Chapter 2 Appendix. The FTC sued the American Medical Association for unfair methods of competition, among them, curtailing physician advertising and not allowing physicians to be paid differential amounts [see Charles D. Weller, "Free Choice as a Restraint of Trade in American Health Care Delivery and Insurance," *Iowa Law Review*, 69 (1984): 1351–1392 for a good description of physician malfeasance].

Chapter 2 Appendix

The American Medical Association, et al. Final Order, Opinion, etc., In Regard to Alleged Violation of the Federal Trade Commission Act

Docket 9064
Final Order, October 12, 1979

On December 19, 1975, the Federal Trade Commission issued its complaint in this matter charging the American Medical Association (AMA), the Connecticut State Medical Society (CSMS), and the New Haven County Medical Association, Inc. (NHCMA) with violations of Section 5 of the Federal Trade Commission Act, 15 U.S.C. 45, by restricting the ability of their members to advertise for and solicit patients and to enter into various contractual arrangements in connection with the offering of their services to the public. Specifically, the complaint charges that respondents have agreed with others to prevent or hinder their members from:

1) Soliciting business, by advertising or otherwise;
2) Engaging in price competition; and
3) Otherwise engaging in competitive practices.

The complaint alleges that respondents and others have caused the agreements to be published and circulated in a publication entitled Principles of Medical Ethics, and they have enforced and abided by the restrictions set forth therein. It is further alleged that, as a result of these acts and practices:

1) Prices of physician services have been stabilized, fixed, or otherwise interfered with;
2) Competition between medical doctors in the provision of such services has been hindered, restrained, foreclosed and frustrated; and
3) Consumers have been deprived of information pertinent to the selection of a physician and of the benefits of competition.

The aforesaid acts, practices and methods of competition are alleged to be unfair and to constitute violations of Section 5 of the Federal Trade Commission Act [2] (p. 706).

A. Organizational Attributes and Acknowledged Benefits to Members

AMA was founded and exists as an organization of and for the medical profession (CX 1042J). The original constitution of AMA proclaimed as one of its purposes, "promoting the usefulness, honor and interests of the medical profession." ... The articles of incorporation adopted by AMA near the turn of the century declared one of its purposes to be "safeguarding the material interests of the medical profession" (CX1355H). In 1975, the AMA House of Delegates recognized that one of the "major missions" of the AMA is to "act as a spokesman for physicians to the public, the government, industry and others" (CX1042S) (p. 741).

• • • • •

Conclusions

I. Factual Summary

The complaint issued in this proceeding challenges the ethics restrictions of respondents AMA, CSMS and NHCMA as violative of Section 5 of the Federal Trade Commission Act, 15 U.S.C. 45. These ethics restrictions do not deal with the medical or therapeutic aspects of a physician's practice; at issue are predominantly restrictions on economic activities. The record evidence presents a substantial body of formal and informal actions initiated, instigated and directly or indirectly influenced by each of the respondents, that have the effect of enhancing the economic positions of the members of each of the respective medical societies. Moreover, this result has not come about through mere chance or coincidence but, rather, through the concerted efforts of each of the respondents and the numerous other constituent (state) and component (local) medical societies located throughout the United States. The end result of their energies has been the placement of a formidable impediment to competition in the delivery of health care services by physicians in this country. That barrier has served to deprive the consumers of the free flow of information about the availability of health care services, to deter the offering of innovative forms of health care and to stifle the rise of almost every type of health care delivery that could potentially pose a threat to the income of fee-for-service physicians in private practice. The costs to the public in terms of less expensive or even, perhaps, more improved medical services are great.

The main body of evidence against respondent AMA consists of the Principles of Medical Ethics, official interpretations of the Principles, which AMA has adopted and disseminated, and letter after letter from AMA officials to medical societies and individual physicians explaining the Principles, applying the Principles to specific conduct and urging compliance with the Principles by the constituent and component societies. This body of evidence, consisting principally of documents from the files of AMA and constituent and component societies located throughout the United States, shows the sweeping nature of the challenged restraints, including a total ban on solicitation of patronage, severe restriction of most forms of advertising and unfair interference with physician's contracts with third parties.

AMA has invited concerted action by its constituents and component medical societies to enforce the challenged restriction. All of AMA's member societies have accepted [233] this role within the AMA ethics framework. They have adopted AMA's Principles of Medical Ethics as their own, their members have abided by them and they have formally and informally enforced the Principles. The Connecticut respondents have adopted AMA's ethical principles and, like AMA's other member societies, have engaged in enforcement of the challenged restrictions (pp. 917–918).

• • • • •

III. Restrictions of Physicians' Advertising, Solicitation and Contractual Relations

A. The Restrictions and their Anticompetitive Effects

Respondent medical societies exercise complete control over physicians' advertising, solicitation and contractual relations. Their control has effectively thwarted competition by physicians in the health care sector. To accomplish these ends, the AMA, CSMS, NHCMA, numerous other constituent and component societies and individual physician members have engaged in a persistent pattern of formal and informal enforcement of broadly based ethics rulings. The means utilized by medical societies in their efforts to perpetuate the fee-for-service physician in private practice and the "usual, customary and reasonable" method of fee reimbursement as the driving forces in medical care in the United States have been the AMA's Principles of Medical Ethics, the AMA Judicial Council Opinions and Reports and sundry interpretations of each. Reliance by the AMA and by constituent and component medical societies upon these sources of ethics pronouncements has been extensive and cannot be disputed in view of the extensive evidence in this record.

Complaints about physician advertising and solicitation often have been submitted to local medical societies, including respondent NHCMA, by individual physicians in the same specialties as the accused doctors. Some of the complaining physicians have expressed concern about the competitive implications of the offending doctors' activities. In response to these complaints, the medical societies have taken restrictive ethics actions regarding the accused physicians. On occasion, they have gone so far as to openly refer to and take into account the competitive concerns expressed by the complaining physicians (pp. 936–937).

• • • • •

IV. Respondents Have Engaged in a Conspiracy to Restrain Competition

The record evidence establishes the existence of a conspiracy between the AMA and its constituent and component medical societies, including respondents CSMS and NHCMA. The degree and pattern of reliance by state and local medical societies upon the AMA for statements of official ethics policy, as well as for advice on ethical matters as they arise or are likely to arise, and the dependence by AMA upon the state and local societies to implement and enforce those ethics policies become manifest in the internal structure and organization of the AMA and its constituent and component societies and in their working interrelationships. The prescriptions and proscriptions of AMA, as set forth in AMA's Principles of Medical Ethics, Judicial Council Opinions and Reports and other official pronouncements represent a pervading force in virtually all disciplinary actions undertaken by medical societies. To conclude, from respondents' admissions and from the parallelism between the nature of official policy on ethical issues as articulated by the AMA and as implemented and enforced by AMA member medical societies, that the striking uniformity of medical societies' positions [280] on ethics matters should have come about by mere chance or coincidence, as respondents have argued, rather than based on a common understanding and concerted activity is to adopt the impractical and ignore the reality (pp. 956–957).

Order

I

It is ordered, that respondents American Medical Association, Connecticut State Medical Society and New Haven County Medical Association, Inc., and their delegates, trustees, councils, committees, officers, representatives, agents, employees, successors and assigns, directly or indirectly, or through any corporate or other device, in or in connection with the purchase, sale, distribution or delivery of physicians' services in or affecting commerce, as "commerce" is defined in the Federal Trade Commission Act, do forthwith cease and desist from:

A. Restricting, regulating, impeding, declaring unethical, interfering with, or advising against the advertising or publishing by any person of the prices, terms or conditions of sale of physicians' services, or of information about physicians' services, facilities or equipment which are offered for sale or made available by physicians or by any organization with which physicians are affiliated;

B. Restricting, regulating, impeding, declaring unethical, interfering with, or advising against the solicitation through [301] advertising or by any other means, of patients, patronage, or contracts to supply physicians' services, by any physician or by any organization with which physicians are affiliated;

C. Restricting, regulating, impeding, advising on the ethical propriety of, or interfering with the commercial terms or conditions on which any physician contracts or seeks to contract for the sale, purchase or distribution of his or her professional services;

D. Restricting, interfering with, or impeding the growth, development or operations of any prepaid health care delivery plan or of any other organization which offers physicians' services to the public, by means of any statement or other representation concerning the ethical propriety of their operations, activities, or relationships with physicians; and

E. Inducing, urging, encouraging, or assisting any physician, or any medical association, group of physicians, hospital [302] insurance carrier or any other nongovernmental organization to take any of the actions prohibited by Paragraphs A through D above. Provided, however, that nothing in this Order shall be construed to prohibit respondents, their constituent or component organizations or their members from reporting in good faith to governmental authorities any alleged violation of law, including but not limited to:

(1) Reporting to appropriate governmental authorities any advertising, solicitation or representation by a physician which they have a reasonable basis for believing is false or deceptive, along with the basis for such belief;

(2) Reporting to appropriate governmental authorities any case of uninvited, in-person solicitation of actual or potential patients who because of their special circumstances are vulnerable to harassment or duress. Provided, further, that after this Order has become final for two years, nothing herein shall prohibit respondents from formulating, adopting and [303] disseminating to their constituent and component medical organizations and to their members ethical guidelines governing the conduct of their members in respect to advertising and solicitation activities, if respondents first obtain permission from and approval of the guidelines by the Federal Trade Commission (pp. 975–976).

• • • • •

This decision was affirmed by an equally divided Supreme Court [455 US 676 (1982)].

3
Hospital Industry

The hospital industry accounts for the largest percentage of dollars spent in the health care sector. In 1995, $350.1 billion was spent on hospital care, although hospital care as a percentage of health care expenditures declined from 47.3 percent in 1980 to 39.8 percent in 1995 (review Table 1-1). As expenses per inpatient day rose from $245 in 1980 to $967 in 1995 [American Hospital Association, *Hospital Statistics*, 1996–1997, Table 1, p. 2], managed care firms in the private sector and Medicare and Medicaid in the public sector have had incentives to keep people out of the hospital.

Unique Characteristics of the Hospital Industry

The administrative management of hospitals may not have the complete control of input costs that management has in most other industries. Jeffrey Harris has suggested that physicians are responsible for patient care and may pay little attention to the costs of care ["The Internal Organization of Hospitals: Some Economic Implications," *Bell Journal of Economics*, 8 (1977): 467–482]. Hospital administrative management cannot control these costs as can manufacturing management control costs of supplies, for example. Recently, however, because of overall hospital cost containment policies of managed care firms, hospital managers have attempted to control physician costs to a much greater extent, for example, by paying physicians a capitated rate for services performed. Physician peer review has been used to question physicians who may treat patients in a more costly manner. Nevertheless, controlling physician costs must be balanced against legal malpractice constraints, which may compel physicians to ignore costs of treatment in caring for patients.

Information on the quality of individual hospitals is far from complete. Hospital care is complex, but other goods and services that are complex have proxy agents or information experts who help consumers evaluate quality. For example, real estate agents help identify and evaluate various

27

homes for customers. Stockbrokers evaluate the stock and bond market for clients. As we have seen, however, in Chapter 2, physicians, as agents for their patients, recommend hospitals and admit patients but may not have enough information or may recommend only those hospitals in which they have staff privileges.

Of hospitals in 1995, 88 percent were nonprofit [American Hospital Statistics, 1996–1997, Table 1, pp. 2–3]. The large percentage of nonprofit hospitals may also indicate that hospitals act differently from other firms. Richard G. Frank and David S. Salkever ["Nonprofit Organizations in the Health Sector," *Journal of Economic Perspectives*, 8 (Fall 1994): 129–144] suggest that nonprofit hospitals may have provided a "trust" signal, given the lack of information on hospital care; there do not appear to be significant differences, however, between nonprofit and for-profit hospitals in providing uncompensated care to hospitalized patients. Moreover, Frank and Salkever suggest that the "trust" signal is disappearing as managed care plans are the buyers who choose hospitals. It is possible, however, that hospitals still receive a derived demand from patients, since patients may select managed care plans based, in part, on their hospital affiliations.

Finally, unlike television sets or video cassette recorders, hospitals appear to be a merit good inasmuch as many believe that individuals are entitled to at least a minimal level of health care services regardless of their ability to pay. Most city, state, and federal laws mandate that hospitals, for example, must provide emergency care to all who seek it.

Changes in the Structure of the Hospital Industry

Horizontal Changes in Structure

A horizontal change in an industry is a change in the number of firms in an industry. For example, a merger between Chrysler Corporation and Ford Motor Corporation would reduce the number of firms that manufacture automobiles. Between 1980 and 1991, there were 195 horizontal hospital mergers (between two or more hospitals) involving 404 hospitals ["AHA Lists Hospital Merger Activity for 12-Year Period," *Hospitals*, June 20, 1992, p. 62]. In part, these mergers may have occurred to make hospitals more efficient. Most studies have found economies of scale in hospitals with approximately 200 beds [see, for example, Carson W. Bays, "The Determinants of Hospital Size: A Survivor Analysis," *Applied Economics* 18 (1986): 359–377], but a recent study suggests that hospitals with fewer than 100 beds may effectively be able to compete in the marketplace [John Simpson, "A Note on Entry by Small Hospitals," *Journal of Health Economics*, 14 (1995): 107–113]. Simpson cites recent evidence from California, which shows that the majority of the twenty general acute care hospitals that opened between January 1989 and March 1993 had fewer than 100 licensed beds, although there is no evidence presented on the length of time these hospitals continued to remain in the market.

Mergers may also occur to achieve monopoly power in a geographic area. It is easier for fewer hospitals to collude and charge monopoly prices. Some mergers may attain monopoly power and also achieve economies of scale. The trade-off between the potential lower costs of economies of scale and the exercise of monopoly power is examined in the antitrust litigation *U.S.* v. *Carilion Health System*, 1989, and *U.S.* v. *Rockford Memorial Corp.*, 1989, provided in the Appendix to this chapter. Hospitals may also merge in order to improve the quality of care they deliver. Evidence suggests that hospitals that perform a greater number of surgeries, for example, may achieve improved quality of care [Harold S. Luft et al., "Should Operations be Regionalized? The Empirical Relation between Surgical Volume and Mortality," *New England Journal of Medicine*, 301 (1979): 1364–1369].

The result of mergers (as well as hospital closings) has been a substantial decline in the number of hospitals in the United States. In 1995, there were 5,220 nonfederal, short-term hospitals in the United States compared to 5,904 hospitals in 1980 and 5,979 in 1975 [American Hospital Association, *Hospital Statistics*, 1996–97, Table 1, p. 2]. Hospital occupancy rates declined from 78 percent in 1980 to 66 percent in 1995.

There has also been a growth of multihospital systems, which may decrease average costs of administration. In 1996, 233 not-for-profit hospital chains owned 1,274 not-for-profit hospitals in the United States, while 45 for-profit chains owned 832 for-profit hospitals ["Statistics for Multihospital Health Care Systems and their Hospitals," *American Hospital Association Hospital Statistics*, 1996–97, p. B53].

Vertical Changes in Structure

A vertical change in structure alters the ownership stages of production of a good or service. For example, if U.S. Steel were to merge with General Motors, the input of steel and the output of an automobile would be vertically integrated into a single firm. The vertical structures of most hospitals have changed, especially since the beginning of the 1990s. Hospitals have merged with physicians or physician groups to form physician-hospital organizations (PHOs). Primary care physician services, for example, may be thought of as input into a second stage of production, such as specialty care or hospitals, to produce health services output. A 1994 Deloitte and Touche and *Hospitals and Health Networks* survey suggests that 71 percent of 1,143 hospitals and 41 health care systems belong to or are developing integrated delivery systems ["The Fading Stand-Alone Hospital," *Hospitals and Health Networks*, June 20, 1994, p. 28]; 24 percent of the respondents in the survey already belonged to a vertically integrated system.

According to a survey performed for the Prospective Payment Assessment Commission in 1993, 15 percent of all hospitals were involved in physician-hospital organizations, including 18 percent of all voluntary, 15 percent of all proprietary, and 9 percent of all government hospitals [Prospective Payment Assessment Commission, *Medicare and the American Health Care System*, Report to Congress, June 1995, Table 4-6, p. 103]. Under this form of vertical integration, hospitals may want to obtain a steadier stream of patients to avoid losing market share. In addition, physician-hospital organizations may achieve some efficiencies in reducing costs of attracting referrals and contracting with managed care plans. The risks of higher-than-expected utilization may be shared between physicians and hospitals.

Thus far, there is no evidence that hospitals that have integrated have realized any economies from integration, such as a reduction in transactions costs. Oliver E. Williamson suggests that the costs of transactions such as contract negotiation and shopping for the best price between two nonintegrated firms may not be insignificant [*Markets and Hierarchies: Analysis and Antitrust Implications* (New York: The Free Press, 1975)]. Physician-hospital organizations may also provide reduced transactions costs for managed care plans that would like to contract with hospitals and physicians. In turn, contracting with managed care plans would potentially achieve higher occupancy rates of hospitals and more physician members of the PHO. This benefit may have to be balanced against cost-reducing competition that managed care firms may engender. A single integrated network may curtail entry of managed care plans and other physicians by limiting hospital staff privileges to its own physicians or by physicians refusing to deal with other managed care plans ["Illegal Price-Fixing Charged in Danbury Hospital Suit," *New York Times*, September 14, 1995, p. B6].

How Do Hospitals Compete?

Competition among hospitals varies depending on the geographic and product markets in which hospitals are located. In metropolitan markets, where there are usually a large number of hospitals, hospitals may compete on a monopolistic competitive basis. Competition may be on a price and nonprice basis. It is also possible that collusion among hospitals takes place. In rural markets, competition may take the form of oligopolistic rivalry, where only a few firms exist. There may be only a single firm dictated by economies of scale and a low population base. The geographic market depends on the degree that prospective patients will substitute one hospital for another (termed the cross-elasticity of demand). Cross-elasticity of demand is defined technically as the percentage change in quantity of hospital services (such as surgical hip or knee replacement) demanded of hospital A divided by the percentage change in the price of these services

Cross elasticity

of hospital B. Cross-elasticity measures the degree to which consumers may switch from one hospital to another in response to a relative change in the price of hospital services. If the cross-elasticity coefficient is greater than 1.0, it is termed elastic; if it is exactly 1.0, it is termed unitary; if less than 1.0, it is termed inelastic.

Cross-elasticity of supply, the percentage change in quantity of services supplied by hospital A divided by the percentage change in the price of these services of hospital B, is similarly important in defining geographic markets. Cross-elasticity of supply attempts to measure the degree of difficulty that competitors might have in entering particular geographic markets. The coefficients may be interpreted in the same way as those that measure cross-elasticity of demand.

In practice, elasticity coefficients are generally not easily calculated since the formula requires that all other possible changes that affect utilization (such as quality) remain constant. Economists may, therefore, utilize patient origin data in calculating geographic markets. That is, the percentage of individuals who may leave a defined geographic area to seek care and the percentage of individuals from outside the defined geographic area who may seek care from hospitals in a defined geographic area is ascertained. If only a small percentage of individuals leave and a small percentage of individuals enter an area for hospital care, the appropriate geographic market may have been approximately defined [Kenneth G. Elzinga and Thomas F. Hogarty, "The Problems of Geographic Market Delineation in Antimerger Suits," *Antitrust Bulletin* 18 (1973): 45–81]. In addition, economists may also examine where physicians have staff privileges and whether there are geographic impediments, such as extensive travel distances, to a geographic market.

After a geographic market is calculated, a hospital product must be established in order to ascertain the degree of competition. Community hospitals may not provide the same services as university hospitals. Eye surgery performed in one hospital does not compete with orthopedic surgery in another hospital. Outpatient services may not compete with inpatient services. Surgicenters may or may not compete with hospitals for some services.

To ascertain the product markets in which hospitals compete, one should again examine the cross-elasticity of demand and supply among possible competing services and among hospitals themselves. Patterns of service use for individuals at different hospitals with different illnesses may be the most helpful.

Hospitals compete on a number of different dimensions. First, hospitals may compete on the amount and types of technology they utilize. With newer, more advanced technology, it might be expected that physicians would be motivated to send a greater number of patients to the hospital. Under this form of competition, one might expect that the greater number of hospitals in an area, the higher the costs [David S. Salkever, "Competition Among Hospitals," in Warren Greenberg, ed., *Competition in the Health Care Sector: Past, Present, and Future*, (Germantown Maryland: Aspen System Corporation, 1978), pp. 149–162]. Competition of this type is perhaps found most often when the third-party payors are predominantly passive insuring organizations who are willing to pay whatever hospital charges for whatever the utilization or technology used.

With the virtual demise of passive insuring organizations and the advent of managed care plans, many hospitals may still compete, in part, on acquiring the latest technology, but prices of hospital services become an element of competition as they are in other industries. Indeed, using Medicare data from as early as 1977–1978, Noether found that lower concentration of hospitals in standard metropolitan statistical areas (SMSAs) is associated with both increased price and quality competition [Monica Noether, "Competition Among Hospitals," *Journal of Health Economics*, 7 (1988): 259–284]. Later evidence from California suggests a hospital marketplace that responds to traditional demand and supply elements. Glenn A. Melnick et al. found that more hospital competition in an area leads to lower hospital prices ["The Effects of Market Structure and Bargaining Position on Hospital Prices," *Journal of Health Economics*, 11 (1992): 217–233].

Melnick et al. hypothesize that the less important the hospital is to a managed care plan (in terms of market share), the lower the price that can be demanded by the managed care plan. If price is too high and there is little patient loyalty to the hospital, the hospital will lose market share. In contrast, Melnick et al. theorize that the lower the market share of the managed care plan the ability to negotiate lower prices is diminished, since an important variable, volume, cannot be used as an enticement to achieve price concessions from providers. Finally, price concessions will be largest where there is greater consumer loyalty to the managed care plan. With consumer loyalty to a managed care plan, a hospital might accept price concessions rather than risk losing the enrollees of the managed care plan [Melnick et al., p. 220].

There has been very little hospital competition based on the perceived quality of hospitals. [For a different view, see Harold S. Luft et al., "Does Quality Influence Choice of Hospital?" *Journal of the American Medical Association*, 263 (1990): 2899–2906]. Competition based on quality has been discouraged by the hospital industry. The Joint Committee on Accreditation of Healthcare Organizations (JCAHO), created by hospitals, accredited more than 99 percent of 1,750 hospitals surveyed in 1994 ["Medical Errors Bring Calls for Change," *New York Times*, July 18, 1995, p. C8] and has yet to issue a report on the perceived quality of individual hospitals. Mortality rates in the United States were published by the U.S. Health Care Financing Administration in 1987–1989 and 1991 for each hospital as a whole and for sixteen high- and low-risk medical conditions. Among these conditions were severe acute heart disease, pulmonary disease, renal disease, low-risk heart disease, and ophthalmic diseases. Mortality rates as a measure of hospital quality, however, have been subject to the criticism that they have not been adjusted accurately. Hospitals that have a sicker patient base may have higher mortality rates even though they provide higher quality care [David W. Smith et al., "Using Clinical Variables to Estimate the Risk of Patient Mortality," *Medical Care*, 29 (1991): 1108–1119]. In addition, many consumers, hospitals, and peer review organizations find the data to be cumbersome and difficult to interpret ["HCFA's Medicare Mortality Data: The Controversy Continues," *Hospitals*, July 5, 1992, pp. 118–122]. The number of procedures performed have been correlated with better outcomes, but a question remains whether number of procedures is a measure of quality or perceived quality. [Harold S. Luft et al., "Should Operations be Regionalized? The Empirical Relation between Surgical Volume and Mortality," *New England Journal of Medicine*, 301 (1979): 1364–1369].[1]

Does the dearth of information published on the quality of hospitals in itself have an effect on the quality of hospital care? One outcome may be that without information on quality some individuals will seek care at suboptimal hospitals. In their study of open-heart surgery, R. H. Kennedy et al. found that 55 percent of all hospitals did fewer than the recommended number of 200 cardiac surgeries a year ["Cardiac-Catheterization and Cardiac-Surgical Facilities," *New England Journal of Medicine*, 307 (1982): 986–992]. If instead more individuals go to "better" hospitals, mortality may decrease and costs may decline because of economies of scale. It is also possible that hospitals will have reduced incentives (except for professional norms) to improve quality of care (since it is not easily measured) and will instead concentrate on attempts to improve areas that are more easily observed. Thus, hospitals might invest in fancy reception areas, general appearance, and smiling reception clerks rather than quality care that improves and lengthens life [George A. Akerlof, "The Market for 'Lemons': Quality Uncertainty and the Market Mechanism," *Quarterly Journal of Economics*, 84 (August 1970): 488–500]. Thus, unless we have good and dependable measures of quality for individual hospitals, the quality of all hospitals may decline. A recent example may be found in the state of New York, where, since 1991, surgeon-specific death rates for coronary bypass surgery have been published. Apparently, 21 of 154 cardiac surgeons have been forced out of the state because of poor records. Moreover, surgeons at one hospital had high mortality rates because patients were not adequately stabilized prior to surgery. Changes in stabilization policy subsequently implemented by the hospital led to reductions in the mortality rates of the

---

[1] Can evaluating hospitals be more complex than evaluating churches and synagogues? *Madison Magazine* in Madison, Wisconsin, attempted to rate churches and synagogues with up to four crosses or stars as well as descriptive paragraphs. Ratings were based on ambience, spirituality, and spiritual leadership [Joe Schoenmann, "The View from the Pew," *Madison Magazine*, December 1994, pp. 52–56].

34   3. Hospital Industry

surgeons ["Death-Rate Rankings Shake New York Cardiac Surgeons," *New York Times*, September 6, 1995, p. 1].

How can more information be produced in the marketplace? The government could resume its publication of mortality rates and at the same time seek to refine and improve the calculations. A list of the hospitals at which a physician has staff privileges could be provided to patients when they first visit the physician. Finally, managed care plans could provide more information on the hospitals belonging to their network. However, as Chapter 11 shows, managed care plans have little incentive to advertise quality.

David Dranove, William D. White, and Lawrence Wu, using hospital patient data from California for 1983 and 1989, found that individuals enrolled in Medicaid more often go to hospitals that offer fewer services ["Segmentation in Local Hospital Markets," *Medical Care*, 31 (1993): 52–64]. Patients in general prefer local hospitals unless they have time to search for the hospital of their choice [p. 64]. However, the authors suggest a potential drawback of increased information: selective contracting would be less effective if everyone with a serious illness wanted to go to the "best" hospital within a geographic area. This hospital would then be able to charge a price commensurate with its superior quality as it differentiates its product. If this becomes the case, the wealthiest individuals will receive the highest-quality care as the "highest quality" is rationed by price. Alternative ways which care may be rationed are discussed in Chapter 10.

Recent Performance of Hospitals

Recent performance of hospitals is evidently akin to what one would expect in traditional microeconomics [David Dranove, Mark Shanley, and William D. White, "Price and Concentration in Hospital Markets: The Switch from Patient-Driven to Payer-Driven Competition," *Journal of Law and Economics*, April 1993, pp. 179–204]. Based on the California selective contracting program from 1983 to 1988, they found that the greater the number of hospitals, the lower the prices and the lower the price-cost margins of the hospitals. This study examines only in-patient treatment of privately insured patients for only a single state, but it provides evidence that traditional economic market models may be an important predictor of hospital behavior and performance. Other evidence suggests that hospitals behave according to economic theory. Michael A. Morrisey's analysis finds evidence of hospitals charging different prices to different payors based on elasticity of demand [*Cost Shifting in Health Care*, (Washington, DC: AEI Press, 1994)]. With this pricing behavior, termed price discrimination, each hospital, with some degree of market power, maximizes its total profit by charging different prices to different payors for the same service. Airlines, for example, maximize profits by charging higher prices for the business person who makes reservations at the last minute in order to sign an important contract, an inelastic demand, and lower prices on the weekend for the college student who might substitute bus or train transportation, an elastic demand.

Health Care Marketplace

As with mergers in any industrial market, when hospitals merge there is often a trade-off between the benefits of economies of scale and the potential cost of higher prices. The benefit-cost ratio of mergers is determined by the degree of competition among hospitals, the nonprofit goals of some hospitals, the geographic and product areas in which hospitals may compete, and the height of any barriers to entry. In *U.S.* v. *Carilion Health System* (1989), the District Court ruled that Carilion was not in violation of the antitrust laws even though the two largest hospitals in a three-hospital market area had merged to form the system. The nonprofit nature of both hospitals seemed to weigh heavily in the court's opinion. In addition, some modest economies of scale were found.

In contrast, in *U.S.* v. *Rockford Memorial Corp.* (1989), where the two largest hospitals in a six-hospital market area merged, the court found a violation of antitrust laws, in part because of high barriers to entry in the form of certificate-of-need laws. The nonprofit status of the hospitals and some economies of scale were given lesser weight. In *Rockford*, the court's ruling was consistent with the industrial organization paradigm that fewer firms would yield higher prices, absent any offsetting economies of scale. With the large increases in number of managed care plans as informed buyers, it is likely that most courts would take this traditional industrial organization view of the industry in the future.

Chapter 3 Appendix

United States of America, Plaintiff,
v.
Carilion Health System and Community Hospital of Roanoke Valley, Defendants

Civ. A. No. 88-0249-R
United States District Court,
W.D. Virginia,
Roanoke Division
Decided February 13, 1989

This antitrust action, brought by the U.S. Justice Department's Antitrust Division to prevent the merger of two hospitals in Roanoke, Virginia, is before the court for entry of judgment. Based on the findings of fact to follow, the court concludes that the government has failed to prove that the planned merger of the defendants would constitute an unreasonable restraint of trade under the antitrust laws and will enter judgment for the defendants (p. 841).

At trial, the government contended that defendants' combination would eliminate actual and potential competition between the two defendants and would lessen competition generally to provide acute inpatient services in the Roanoke Valley (p. 841).

Defendant Carilion Health System is a nonstock, nonprofit holding company that owns three nonprofit hospitals in Virginia and manages six others. The company also owns a number of for-profit subsidiaries, including a helicopter ambulance service, an eye, ear, nose and throat clinic, a pharmacy, an insurance company and a health club. Carilion's largest facility is Roanoke Memorial Hospital in Roanoke, a facility licensed by Virginia health planning authorities for 677 acute inpatient beds, of which the hospital staffs and operates 609. Occupancy averages something less than 500 patients. Roanoke Memorial is a teaching affiliate for the University of Virginia Medical School in Charlottesville. . . .

Defendant Community Hospital of Roanoke Valley is a nonstock, nonprofit corporation that owns a hospital by the same name in downtown Roanoke. The facility has 400 licensed beds of which 220 are staffed. Occupancy averages about 175 patients. Both Carilion and Community have been organized principally to provide hospital services to the general public, and both provide indigent care to the extent that funds are available. The boards of directors of both institutions are comprised in large part of business leaders from the Roanoke area who have sought to minimize health care costs to employers and patients.

Both Roanoke Memorial and Community draw more than half their patients from the Roanoke metropolitan area, including the cities of Roanoke and Salem and Roanoke County. About 53 percent of Roanoke Memorial's patients come from this area, while Community draws about 74 percent of its patients from there. If defendants' planned affiliation took place, a third facility in the Roanoke area, Lewis-Gale Hospital in Salem, would not be involved in the transaction. Owned by Hospital Corporation of America, Lewis-Gale is licensed for 406 beds, of which it operates about 335. The hospital's average occupancy is about 242. Lewis-Gale receives about 70 percent of its patients from the Roanoke area (p. 842).

All three of these hospitals draw substantial numbers of patients from outside the immediate vicinity of Roanoke (p. 843).

All three of the hospitals in Roanoke and Salem provide primary, secondary and some types of tertiary care (p. 843).

About 20 other hospitals within the geographic area Roanoke Memorial and, to some extent, Community serve provide primary and, in some cases, secondary level services (p. 843).

[F]acts show that the Roanoke hospitals compete with the various hospitals in the counties that surround Roanoke to provide primary and secondary level care to patients from those areas (p. 844).

In providing tertiary care, the Roanoke hospitals do not face competition from the hospitals in surrounding counties, but several other large hospitals in Virginia and North Carolina do compete with them (p. 844).

New entry into the hospital market would be financially difficult. Expansion of an existing hospital, however, would cost substantially less.... However, most hospitals now staff substantially fewer beds than their licensed capacity and could expand to their full licensed quotas without obtaining state approval. Moreover, the number of problems treated on an inpatient basis has declined steadily in recent years and can be expected to continue to fall. Defendants' hospitals and their competitors can therefore be expected to have even more beds to fill within their licensed capacity, and competition for patients can therefore be expected to intensify further. And even if state ceilings did limit a hospital's capacity to accept more patients, it appears likely that Virginia will soon remove its caps on the number of beds hospitals can have.... Virginia's Secretary of Health and Human Resources, firmly predicted at trial that Virginia would soon follow the lead of other states in deregulating the hospital industry (p. 845).

Under defendants' planned affiliation, which defendants approved on July 30, 1987, Carilion would acquire sole membership in and ownership of

Community, and Community would gain minority representation on Carilion's board of directors. Defendants want to merge in order to enhance the competitive positions of both Roanoke Memorial and Community. Roanoke Memorial needs more space in which to offer its obstetrics services and for various other clinical and administrative functions. On the other hand, Community's occupancy has declined faster than that of Roanoke's other hospitals. Community has extra space and needs more patients. Defendants plan to consolidate all obstetrics and other clinical services of both hospitals at Community. The merger also can be expected to help the two hospitals strengthen and expand joint operations, which already have begun in the areas of data processing and laundry. Credible testimony at trial satisfies the court the merger will produce capital avoidance and other clinical and administrative efficiencies that will save the two hospitals at least $40 million over the first five years of the affiliation (pp. 845-846).

Based on expert testimony, the court also finds that as a general rule hospital rates are lower, the fewer the number of hospitals in an area. In addition, charitable, nonprofit hospitals tend to charge lower rates than for-profit hospitals. Relative to other products and services consumers buy, hospital services are not price sensitive in a relevant market. Finally, the Virginia Health Services Cost Review Council can be expected to use effective persuasive power to keep hospital rates relatively low in western Virginia. While the Council's official powers are hortatory, hospitals and the press closely watch its publication of hospital rates (p. 846).

In conclusion, the court finds that the planned merger would probably improve the quality of health care in western Virginia and reduce its cost and will strengthen competition between the two large hospitals that would remain in the Roanoke area. Defendants' boards of directors could be expected to help insure that savings realized from the affiliation will be passed on to consumers (p. 846).

The District Court's opinion was subsequently upheld by the 4th Circuit Court of Appeals [*United States* v. *Carilion Health System*, 892 F.2d 1042; 1989-2 Trade Case (CCH) P68, 859].

United States of America, Plaintiff,
v.
Rockford Memorial Corporation and SwedishAmerican Corporation,

Defendants
No. 88 C20186
United States District Court,
N.D. Illinois, W.D.
Decided February 23, 1989

United States brought action to enjoin proposed consolidation of not-for-profit hospitals as violative of antitrust laws. The District Court ... held that proposed consolidation of not-for-profit hospitals violated [the] antitrust statute prohibiting acquisitions which might effect substantial lessening of competition, and thus would be enjoined, in that merger would result in single hospital controlling almost 70% of geographic market, with two largest hospitals in area increasing their share of area's inpatient hospital business from 64% to 90% (p. 1251)....

The provision of outpatient care by all healthcare providers, including hospitals, is increasing and will continue to do so in the foreseeable future. In hospitals, the same facilities and personnel used to provide inpatient care is also used to provide outpatient care. In addition, many outpatients treated by hospitals are ultimately admitted as inpatients. Undoubtedly, there is direct competition between the individual outpatient services provided by hospitals and nonhospitals (FF ¶¶ 58–65). Despite the presence of this strain of competition, outpatient care is no substitute for acute inpatient hospital care. The outpatient provider represents a few procedures at most and cannot provide in any circumstance, an overnight stay. In providing patient care, the hospital may utilize a procedure that competes directly with outpatient providers when used alone for an outpatient. However, all competition and substitutability between the hospital and the outpatient provider ends when that same outpatient procedure is used in tandem with other services to treat an inpatient. The outpatient provider has nothing comparable to offer (FF ¶¶ 66–67) (p. 1261).

If the defendants could assert a small but significant and nontransitory price increase in inpatient care, the exercise of market power could not be ameliorated by outpatient care. Of course, there are some inpatients currently receiving inpatient care that could possibly utilize outpatient care, but not in numbers significant enough to break an exercise of market power in the inpatient care market (p. 1261).

It is true, as the defendants contend, that nonhospital providers such as outpatient clinics, emergency care centers, doctors offices and other providers, offer some of the same services as do acute care hospitals. Furthermore, it is also true that the relevant product market must include all services provided by acute care hospitals and those services offered by nonhospital providers which are an alternative to hospital care. However, only the acute care hospitals can provide the unique combinations of services which an acute care patient must have. Outpatient facilities routinely feed patients to the hospitals' inpatient facilities. Those services include both inpatient and outpatient care, both of which are competed for by acute care hospitals. Accordingly, the court finds that the relevant product market consists of that cluster of services offered only by acute care hospitals . . . (p. 1261).

The government explains that hospital admissions are determined, for the most part, not by putative inpatients but by their physicians. These physicians will invariably admit patients to hospitals where the physicians have admitting privileges. In turn, physicians seek admitting privileges at hospitals where they anticipate admitting a significant number of their patients. Usually, physicians want to admit patients to institutions that are convenient both to themselves and their patients. Doctors favor hospitals close enough to allow them to conduct their daily practice and still have time to check patients on daily rounds and if need be to respond quickly to an inpatient in need of immediate attention. In this same vein, patients generally desire to be admitted to a hospital near their family and friends and their admitting physician. In sum, physicians and patients generally choose to use relatively close hospitals (FF ¶¶ 68–73) (p. 1262).

The government argues that this tendency for convenience in admitting significantly limits the number of competitors in the market. The government points to the fact that of the approximately 450 physicians in the "Rockford area" nearly all of them have admitting privileges, either active or courtesy, with all three Rockford area hospitals (RMH, SAH and STA) [Rockford Memorial Hospital, Swedish-American Hospital, St. Anthony Hospital] but nowhere else. Thus, if a "Rockford area" physician's patient wanted to stay at a hospital other than RMH, STA or SAH, he or she would need to be referred to a non-Rockford physician to admit him or her (Tr. 130, 517, pp. 1268–1269). The government surmises that these admitting patterns show that doctors in the "Rockford area" are unwilling to admit their regular patients to hospitals outside the "Rockford area," forcing them to travel longer distances to fulfill their duties. The government further concludes that these same doctors will be unwilling to give up the convenience of the nearby Rockford hospitals for others farther away, even in the event of a price increase in inpatient care at the defendants' hospitals (pp. 1262–1263).

Similarly, the government points out that another important group, third party payers, also prefer nearby hospitals. These payers are not amenable to purchasing healthcare outside the three Rockford hospitals for "Rockford area" patients (FF ¶ 80). Third party payers are employers, Medicare,

Medicaid, and healthcare indemnity insurers such as Blue Cross and Aetna. These payers are the true purchasers of healthcare in most instances. In addition, managed health care plans such as Health Maintenance Organizations ("HMO") and Preferred Provider Organizations ("PPO") are involved in purchasing healthcare. A HMO contracts with a group of physicians to perform medical services for plan subscribers at a set prepaid fee. A PPO is an agreement between a health provider such as a hospital or clinic and a purchaser. The agreement usually consists of the provider granting a discount to purchasers in return for the purchaser's promise to send patients to the health provider (FF ¶¶ 75–79). Based on the same doctor/patient sentiment for convenience outlined above, these third party payers are wary of attempting to force plan beneficiaries from their local Rockford hospitals to relatively distant hospitals (FF ¶¶ 75–80) (p. 1263).

In sum, the court has arrived at an area where the defendants compete with four other hospitals for the group of patients representing about 90% of the admissions of the defendants. Any area greater would be unrealistic in that competitors in those areas do not compete to any significant extent for the same patients as the defendants. Any area smaller would ignore competitors who, while small, do compete for a significant segment of the defendants' admission base (p. 1278).

Further, the merger reduces the number of competitors in the market from 6 to 5. Although this reduction from 6 to 5 appears rather innocuous, the merger eliminates the competition between the two largest competitors in the market, however defined (i.e. beds, patient days, admissions). If the affiliation of St. Anthony with St. Joseph and Swedish-American with Highland is factored into the market share determination, then the merged entity accounts for 70.4% (beds), 71.7% (admissions), and 75.3% (inpatient days) share of the post-merger relevant market (DX 101). The merger then would reduce the number of competitors in the market from 4 to 3 (p. 1280).

. . . it is necessary to measure the relative ease or difficulty of entering the relevant market.

In the instant case, a new entrant must overcome regulatory barriers to enter the relevant market. The Illinois Certificate-of-Need law presents a formidable barrier to persons wishing to provide new acute hospital inpatient care in the WOB area. Before a provider adds new bed capacity, purchases capital equipment worth more than four hundred thousand dollars or changes services offered, a certificate-of-need (CON) must be obtained from the Illinois Health Facility Planning Board, a state body (Tr. 425–426) (p. 1281).

The first burden placed on a potential market entrant (i.e., a new acute care hospital) by the CON is the expense and length of the CON application process. While the initial application process itself may take some time, historically the biggest delays occur when competing hospitals challenge the granting of a CON and/or an applicant who is originally denied a CON appeals to the state courts (see FF ¶¶ 127–130). Moreover, there is no guarantee that a CON will eventually be obtained even after completing the expensive and often arduous application process (GX 25). Consequently, the CON regulation, by definition, serves as a barrier to entry (pp. 1281–1282).

In sum, the defendants have demonstrated that the merger will generate some unique savings, but no more than normal and certainly not enough to override §7 of the Clayton Act. Even if all the defendants' savings were verifiable and could only be achieved through merger, the amount saved pales in comparison to the likely amount of revenues generated by the defendants in the same five year period (Tr. 2069). Moreover, monopoly rents could far outweigh the savings presented, particularly in light of the fact that much of the savings cited by the defendants were not clearly and convincingly generated by the merger. Large amounts of savings could be achieved independent of a merger through alternative action or a drop in production. Moreover, if costs related to the merger are taken into account, even more savings would be offset. This court is not unaware, nor unsympathetic with, the defendants' desire to improve their respective positions by establishing a new, more powerful economic entity. Certainly, viewing the proposed merger from the perspective of a purely business decision, the merger makes sense. It would allow the new entity to eliminate certain duplicative services and equipment, with the attendant reduction in personnel and other costs. It would improve the capital position of the new entity, as opposed to the old entities, thus allowing for greater expenditures for equipment and possibly improving the ability of the new entity to buy in larger quantities, reducing some costs. It might also allow the new entity to improve its services to the extent that it might become a major medical center, providing tertiary care in a wider range of services and in a broader geographical area. These are but a few of the business advantages which may inure to the benefit of the defendants if the merger is allowed to proceed. Others may also come to mind. In an antitrust context, however, it is *competition*, not the *competitors*, which the laws seek to protect. See *Brown Shoe*, 370 U.S. at 320, 82 S.Ct. at 1521. If the court's task was motivated by the same business and economic considerations as those of the defendants, the inquiry could end here (p. 1291).

The District Court's opinion was subsequently upheld by the 7th Circuit Court of Appeals [*United States* v. *Rockford Memorial Corporation*, 898 F.2d 1278, 1282 (7th Circuit) *cert. Denied*, 498 U.S. 920 (1990)].

4
Insurance, Managed Care, and System Integration

Approximately two-thirds of all health care expenditures are paid for by insurance. In contrast, purchases of other goods and services involve only a buyer and a seller, with no intermediate payor. As the intermediate payor, the insuring organization is the fulcrum around which the health care industry turns. In this chapter I review the reasons why insurance is so pervasive in the health care sector and why insurance for health care expenditures is usually different than insurance for other goods and services. The effects of insurance on prices and health services delivered are shown. The focus of this chapter is on the structure, behavior, and performance of insuring organizations and their effects on competition in the health insurance market. I analyze system integration and close the chapter with an examination of the status of the uninsured in the United States.

Insurance in the Health Care Sector

Insurance is generally purchased when there is the possibility of random, costly occurrences. Automobile accidents or fire involving one's property are such events. People prefer to pay a predictable monthly or annual premium rather than the entire cost at one time for these random events. Health insurance is also bought to guard against unpredictable occurrences. Health insurance is similar to other kinds of insurance in another way. Insuring organizations, in competition with one another, each have incentives to contain costs.

There is one important difference, however, between health insurance and most other kinds of insurance. Health insurance is subject to moral hazard. Moral hazard is the consumption of a greater amount of services when insurance is available compared to when it is not available. People do not set fire to their homes because they have fire insurance, but people do use more health services when they have health insurance. Studies have shown, for example, that people with complete health insurance coverage consume almost one-third more health services than those with large

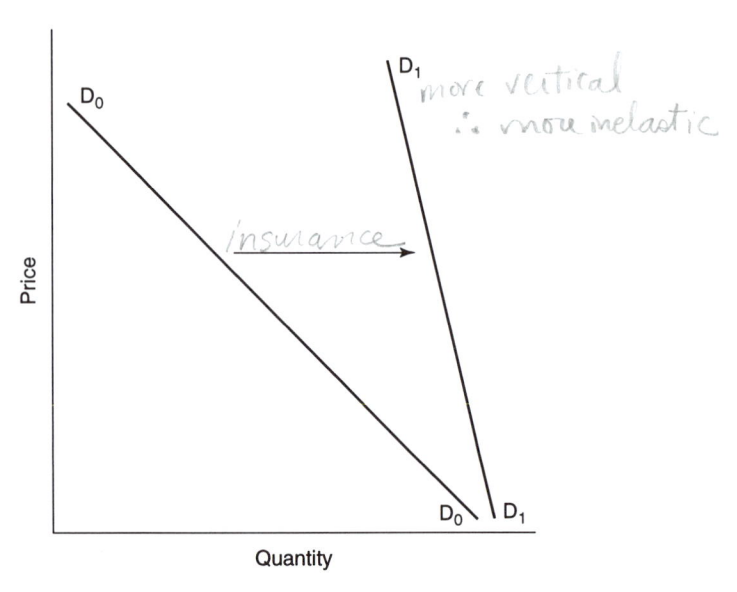

FIGURE 4-1. D₁–D₁, the effect of insurance on demand of health care services

deductibles. In other words, a nonzero price elasticity of demand exists for health care services. Manning and his colleagues, in a major Rand Corporation survey, calculate the price elasticity at approximately −0.2 [Willard G. Manning et al., "Health Insurance and the Demand for Medical Care: Evidence from a Randomized Experiment," *American Economic Review*, 77 (June 1987): 251–277].

The presence of insurance for health care services, therefore, may be at least partially responsible for rising prices and increased use of these services. Insurance shifts the demand curve to the right for health care services, and it makes the demand curve more inelastic. Increased prices and services demanded are shown in Figure 4-1. The extent of the price increase and services demanded depends on the elasticity of demand for the particular health care service. It is not clear, however, that the presence of health insurance leads to better health outcomes. David M. Cutler concludes from his examination of the research evidence that there is not much difference in health outcomes between people with different levels of health insurance or different reimbursement mechanisms ["The Cost and Financing of Health Care," *American Economic Association (AEA) Papers and Proceedings*, May 1995, pp. 32–37].

Blue Cross and Blue Shield

The first Blue Cross plan was created in 1932 by hospitals in order to ensure that they would receive payment for services delivered to their patients.

Individuals prepaid each month and, in turn, the Blue Cross plans reimbursed the hospital for charges when services were delivered. Blue Shield was begun in 1939 by physicians who wanted to ensure payment for their services. In the 1970s, 1980s, and 1990s, many Blue Cross and Blue Shield plans in more than sixty areas throughout the United States merged to become combined Blue Cross and Blue Shield plans.

For forty years, Blue Cross and Blue Shield plans were mostly indemnity, fee-for-service plans, with little cost containment or utilization review aside from the requirements of some plans that second opinions were necessary in order to be reimbursed for elective surgery. Blue Cross and Blue Shield plans also typically insured individuals on a community rating basis. Under community rating, all individuals or groups of individual's are charged the same premium regardless of a single individual's or group's health status. Community rating, therefore, means that healthy individuals subsidize individuals who have the potential of becoming sick or are already ill. As Mark V. Pauly suggests, low-risk individuals buy too little insurance because the price is relatively high, and high-risk individuals buy too much insurance because prices are relatively low ["The Welfare Economics of Community Rating," *Journal of Risk and Insurance*, 37 (1970): 407–418]. On fairness or equity grounds, however, community rating, as opposed to experience rating where each person or group pays a premium equal to its marginal cost, ensures that those with high-cost illnesses are not paying a premium many times greater than those without such illnesses.

Because of its size, Blue Cross and Blue Shield was also able to receive a discount on charges by hospitals. This discount, along with their recognized trade name, helped Blue Cross and Blue Shield keep their dominant positions in health insurance [Roger Feldman and Warren Greenberg, "The Relationship Between Blue Cross Market Share and Blue Cross Discount on Hospital Charges," *Journal of Risk and Insurance*, 48 (1981): 235–246]. Most states regulated the premiums Blue Cross and Blue Shield could set in exchange for the willingness to preserve community rating and to make greater efforts to enroll high-risk individuals.

Blue Cross and Blue Shield has been challenged in the fee-for-service market by approximately 1,300 commercial insurers. Many of these insurers, such as Prudential and Aetna, also provide insurance for property or major life expenses. Typically, the commercials competed with Blue Cross and Blue Shield by experience rating their premiums. Thus, the commercial insurers were able to set their premiums below the Blue Cross and Blue Shield plans for low-risk individuals, although most Blue Cross and Blue Shield plans have resorted to experience rating as well.

Managed Care

Chapter 1 showed that the economics of health care are different from the economics of other goods and services because of information asymmetries and the presence of insurance. The cost-conscious insuring organization or managed care plan modifies these distinctions. Managed care plans have incentives to keep costs low. For example, they can select physicians who practice the least expensive form of medicine. They can choose hospitals that have the lowest rates. Managed care plans may, therefore, reduce the asymmetry of information between providers and the purchasers of care. Managed care plans also have the capability to provide information on the quality of care of providers to potential patients, but Chapter 11 suggests that they have very little incentive to provide this information.

Managed care firms consist of health maintenance organizations (HMOs), preferred provider organizations (PPOs), point-of-service plans (POSs), and various alternative delivery systems, such as competitive medical plans (CMPs), the term used for managed care plans in Medicare, and exclusive provider options (EPOs), which require extremely large out-of-pocket payments when a provider is used outside of the system. The 95 percent of fee-for-service plans that have a utilization review component may even be included in some definitions of managed care. Managed care firms are rationing devices that curtail the utilization and fees of health care services. Managed care organizations may also be defined as organizations that, through economic incentives or actual intervention, affect the level of health care provided to the patient. Under managed care, providers may be at risk for the delivery of services or may undergo utilization review by a third party. Managed care may also mean a restriction in the number of providers in a particular plan. Selecting a provider outside a plan usually results in financial penalties for patients. Some managed care firms employ gatekeepers in order to keep costs controlled. Gatekeepers are usually primary care physicians or nurses whom patients must see first to be referred to higher-cost specialists.

Managed care firms provide coverage for most health care services, including hospitalization and physician care. Some managed care firms, however, specialize in specific areas, such as pharmaceuticals or mental health or substance abuse services. There may be efficiencies to these "carve-outs," but no data are yet available that measure their efficiency.

Health Maintenance Organizations

A health maintenance organization (HMO) is a prepaid health insurance plan in which the organization is responsible for the delivery of health care services. Health maintenance organizations may be divided into four different models, staff, group, network, and individual practice associations (IPA).

Staff model HMOs pay employed physicians on a salary basis. Group model HMOs contract with an independent group of physicians for health care services. Network HMOs contract with two or more independent groups of physicians. Under group and network model HMOs, physicians may be paid a capitated or flat sum for each patient they see. Finally, IPAs are individual physicians practicing in their own offices who contract with the IPA organization for a capitated or fee-for-service amount. When physicians receive a capitated sum and are at financial risk for their services, they have less incentive to see patients or to perform additional services. In addition, when physicians are paid a salary, they have no incentive to perform as many services as they would in fee-for-service practice.

W. Pete Welch, Alan L. Hillman, and Mark V. Pauly ["Toward New Typologies for HMOs," *Milbank Quarterly*, 68 (1990): 221–243] suggest a characterization of HMOs based on organizational and financial elements. Their characteristics include the methods of payment of physicians, the mix of fee-for-service and HMO patients seen by the physician, the direct or indirect contracts the HMO has with physicians, the extent of the risk that primary care physicians may bear, and the number of physicians in particular risk pools. Each of these characteristics affects the behavior of physicians. For example, physicians who see a greater number of HMO patients may more easily adapt to an HMO-style of practice than those who see a greater number of fee-for-service patients. In 1993, 546 HMOs enrolled nearly 47 million individuals [Health Insurance Association of America, *Source Book of Health Insurance Data*, 1994, Table 2.14, p. 44].

Preferred Provider Organizations

Preferred provider organizations (PPOs) are health care plans that do not include all providers in an area and do not reimburse providers at the same rate. The PPO chooses the providers who will provide the optimum mix of quality and cost to the plan and its potential customers, and they usually pay lower benefits if patients use a provider who is not included in the PPO network. At the beginning of 1993, 895 PPOs enrolled more than 50 million individuals [Health Insurance Association of America, *Source Book of Health Insurance Data*, 1994, Table 2.19, p. 48].

Point-of-Service Plans

Point-of-service plans (POS) are combinations of fee-for-service and HMO plans. An enrollee in a POS can decide just before care is rendered whether it should be obtained from a fee-for-service (at higher prices) or an HMO provider. In this way the enrollee not only chooses a plan but also chooses the treatment format when service is desired. Point-of-service plans are the fastest-growing type of plan. In 1994, there were 349 POSs, an increase of 144 POS plans since 1990 [Group Health Association of America "Enrollment in Point-of-Service (POS) and Administrative Services Only (ASO) Products, Year-End 1994," *1995 National Directory of HMOs*, p. 49].

Self-Insured Plans

A large number of employers have elected to self-insure for health care expenditures rather than retain an insuring organization to spread and pool its risks along with other employers. A major reason for self-insurance is the Employee Retirement Income Security Act of 1974 (ERISA), which prohibits state regulation of self-insured health plans. States, for example, have often regulated and mandated costly health care benefits that may add to an employer's costs [Mary Ann Chirba-Martin and Troyen A. Brennan, "The Critical Role of ERISA in State Health Reform," *Health Affairs*, 11, (1994): 142–156]. More than 50 percent of employees are currently in plans that are self-insured, and about 75 percent of firms with 1,000 or more employees are self-insured [Jonathan P. Weiner and Gregory de Lissovoy, "Razing a Tower of Babel: A Taxonomy for Managed Care and Health Insurance Plans," *Journal of Health Politics, Policy and Law*, 18 (1993): 75–103].

How Do Managed Care Firms Compete?

Managed care firms may compete by containing costs. Randall P. Ellis and Thomas G. McGuire divide cost containment into supply-side and demand-side categories ["Supply-Side and Demand-Side Cost Sharing in Health Care," *Journal of Economic Perspectives*, 7 (Fall 1993): 135–151]. Any prospective payment scheme can be regarded as supply-side cost containment since providers or suppliers are placed at risk [Ellis and McGuire, p. 139]. A fixed capitation rate has the greatest supply-side risk for providers since any services performed that cost more than the capitation rate mean an out-of-pocket loss for the provider. In contrast to demand-side cost containment, the effects of supply-side cost containment do not vary by income status. Demand-side cost containment consists of deductibles or copayments the patient must pay. Evidence suggests that physician visits are reduced, although reductions in hospital lengths of stay are not substantial. Willard G. Manning et al., however, found that total costs can be contained for all health care expenses relative to a plan that pays for full coverage ["Health Insurance and the Demand for Medical Care: Evidence from a Randomized Experiment," *American Economic Review*, June 1987, pp. 251–277]. Demand-side cost containment puts most of the burden on patients, who may have health problems if visits to providers are neglected. Demand-side cost containment also places a greater burden on individuals with lower incomes since they have to pay a greater proportion of their income in copayments and deductibles [Ellis and McGuire, p. 147]. Providers may also experience fewer visits and perhaps realize lower incomes.

Most evidence suggests that managed care plans have been able to contain health care costs to a greater extent than fee-for-service plans without any reduction in quality. Interpretation of the evidence is complex, however, because of the large number of different types of managed care plans as well as differences within each managed care plan, the extent of integration with providers, the difficulties in measuring quality, the different regions of the United States, the amount of competition in an area, the different years of evidence, and the different case mix of individuals within the plans. Moreover, evidence generally concerns controlling one aspect of health care costs, such as hospitalization, without taking into consideration other aspects, such as the utilization of physician services.

Harold S. Luft found that HMOs had lower hospital admission rates than fee-for-service indemnity plans ["How Do Health Maintenance Organizations Achieve Their Savings?" *New England Journal of Medicine*, 298, (1978): 1336–1343]. Robert H. Miller and Luft also found lower hospital admission rates in HMOs compared to indemnity plans ["Managed Care Plan Performance since 1980," *Journal of the American Medical Association*, 271 (1994): pp. 1512–1519]. In addition, HMOs had shorter lengths of stay and fewer hospital days per enrollee relative to fee-for-service plans [p. 1514]. HMO enrollees also had more preventive care and physician office visits, but it is unclear how much prevention contributed to cost containment (pp. 1516, 1517). Miller and Luft conclude from their examination of the literature that "HMOs provide care at lower cost than do indemnity plans," with no decrease in quality [p. 1517].

In general, it appears that staff-model HMOs control costs no better than IPA model HMOs [Miller and Luft, p. 1517]. This may suggest that capitation formulas used in some IPAs have become much more stringent than those prior to the 1978 Luft study. Since the case mix as well as the internal incentives and external environment of plans is constantly changing, it has been difficult to measure the long-run effects of HMOs on cost and quality. Insuring organizations also have incentives to offer preventive health programs in order to contain future health care costs. This incentive may be limited, however, because enrollees can switch to other plans, and the resources spent in preventive care can accrue in the form of lower costs to the new insurer.

Utilization review consists of third-party review of physician admissions and review of lengths of stay in the hospital. Thomas M. Wickizer ["The Effect of Utilization Review on Hospital Use and Expenditures: A Review of the Literature and an Update on Recent Findings, *Medical Care Review*, 47 (1990): 327–363] finds that most of the savings from utilization review stem from reductions of admissions to hospitals (p. 356). Offsetting this reduction in admissions, but to a minor extent, was a significant increase in hospital outpatient care expenditures.

50   4. Insurance, Managed Care, and System Integration

Managed Care Firms and the Use of Monopsony Power

Although managed care plans have incentives to contain costs, it is possible that a managed care firm (or even a traditional insuring organization) with a large market share might drive provider fees below their marginal costs and might also reduce utilization below what would be purchased in a competitive market. Such firms are termed monopsonies, or single-buyer firms. The inefficiencies caused by a monopsony buyer are akin to the inefficiencies created by a monopoly seller.

The consequences of monopsony pricing are shown in Figure 4-2 [see, also, in general, Mark V. Pauly, "Market Power, Monopsony, and Health Insurance Markets," *Journal of Health Economics*, 7 (1988): 111–128]. Note that there is a social loss because firms must purchase each input at the same low price. Moreover, because of these lower costs, the monopsonist might increase its monopoly power over potential rivals.

The possibility of finding a monopsony insuring organization is remote, given that there are few barriers to entry in this marketplace. Blue Cross and Blue Shield had a market share that exceeded 80 percent in the state of Rhode Island in the 1980s due, in part, to their exemption from premium taxes and their nonprofit status. Allegations that they exerted

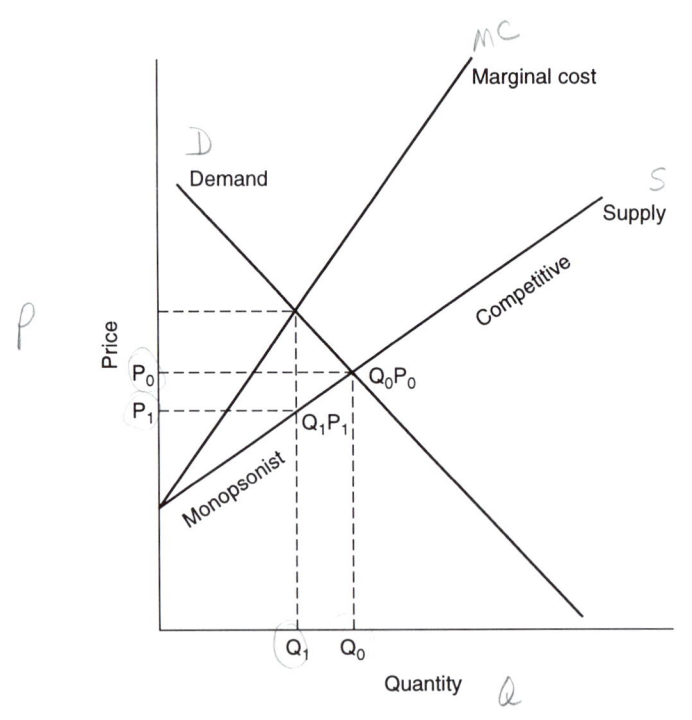

FIGURE 4-2. Monopsony in the health care market. Q_1 quantities are sold at price P_1 ($Q_1 P_1$). In contrast, the competitive price is P_0 and quantity sold is Q_0

monopsonistic power over physicians were denied by the Court of Appeals in an antitrust action brought by a competing health maintenance organization [see the District Court decision in the Appendix to this chapter as well as Chapter 8]. In Rhode Island, participating physicians of Blue Cross were required to sign contracts that prohibited them from accepting lower reimbursement payments from a new, entering insuring organization. This ensured that Blue Cross/Blue Shield would pay the lowest fee for physician services, but it made it more difficult for rivals to enter the market by paying lower fees to physicians [Lawrence G. Goldberg and Warren Greenberg, "The Response of the Dominant Firm to Competition," *Health Care Management Review*, Winter 1995, pp. 65–74]. Often, public policy trade-offs have to be made between the desired goal of cost containment and the potential of monopsonistic pricing and increasing barriers to entry.

Managed Care and Cream Skimming

In addition to incentives to contain costs, managed care firms have incentives to avoid potentially high-risk or high-cost individuals. Evidence of Marc L. Berk and Alan C. Monheit shows that only 1 percent of the population incurred 30 percent of health care costs and only 2 percent of the population incurred 41 percent of health care costs in 1987. In contrast, the bottom 50 percent of the population (in terms of health care costs) incurred only 3 percent of health care costs ["The Concentration of Health Expenditures: An Update," *Health Affairs*, Winter 1992, pp. 145–149]. Each insuring organization, therefore, has enormous incentives to enroll the healthiest people in its area. If people in ill health were to enroll, premiums would rise for everyone in the plan and potential profits would be reduced. As premiums rise, it causes the healthiest individuals to drop out of the plan, which again increases the premiums for those still left in the plan [Michael Rothschild and Joseph Stiglitz, "Equilibrium in Competitive Insurance Markets: An Essay on the Economics of Imperfect Information," *Quarterly Journal of Economics*, 90 (1976): 629–649].

The incentives of managed care firms to avoid high-risk individuals has a number of undesirable effects. First, it affects the ability of health insuring organizations to deliver quality care. If a managed care firm becomes known as a provider of quality health care for all chronically ill patients, for example, it will attract high risk patients in the next enrollment period. Thus, long waits for appointments, difficulties in seeing specialists, and rude personnel may not be uncommon ['Managed Care Has Trouble Treating AIDS, Patients Say," *New York Times*, January 15, 1996, p. A1].

Second, firms that are more efficient in cost containment, in their organizational structure, and in the production of higher quality health care may be put out of business by cream-skimming rivals. Third, if cream skimming is effective, high-risk individuals may be unable to secure health insurance, resulting in a decline in health status and a potential productivity loss if these individuals need medical treatment.

Fourth, managed care firms have reduced incentives to provide increased information about the quality of providers with whom they contract for fear of attracting high-risk individuals. A potential advantage that managed care firms have is the ability to provide increased information on the quality of providers in an area. An organization, however, may find it costly to be known as the managed care firm that uses the best surgeons or has the best tertiary care.

Managed care firms have developed ways to be more attractive to healthy individuals. They may locate, for example, in suburban areas where there is a larger number of young, healthy members and avoid inner-city areas where individuals tend to be in poorer health. They may offer membership in athletic clubs, which would be more appealing to healthy individuals. They may offer high deductibles, which would be less appealing to those with serious illnesses. Fred J. Hellinger, in his compilation of the evidence ["Selection Bias in HMOs and PPOs: A Review of the Evidence," *Inquiry*, 32 (Summer 1995): 135–142], finds that traditional managed care plans that restrict use of provider have a lower-risk population of elderly and nonelderly than fee-for-service plans. Individuals who have been sick or who have chronic conditions are reluctant to leave their own physician in a fee-for-service plan.

Hellinger suggests that it is possible that managed care firms with a smaller network of physicians would have more favorable selection compared to those with larger networks [p. 141]. Consistent with this possibility, Ira Strumwasser et al. ["The Triple Option Choice: Self-Selection Bias in Traditional Coverage, HMOs, and PPOs," *Inquiry*, 26 (Winter 1989): 432–441] found, in a first-time offering of a variety of plans, that given the option of a traditional fee-for-service plan, an HMO, or a PPO, individuals who were previously members of the fee-for-service plan and switched to an HMO or PPO were younger and had lower average expenses as well as lower inpatient and outpatient utilization rates.

Potential Antidotes to Cream Skimming

Competition based on cream skimming leads to the delivery of lower-quality health care, less access to health insurance in general, and little or no insurance for high-risk individuals. A possible solution to cream skimming would be for insurers to experience-rate each applicant and base the premium on the health status of the individual. This is not unlike an automobile insurer charging a higher amount for a teenage male because the probability of accidents among teenage males is much higher than among the rest of the population. In health care, however, societal pressures may make it unacceptable for insuring organizations to charge an AIDS patient, for example, a premium of $50,000 a year or more to cover the costs of treatment.

A second proposal is for the government to mandate that high-risk individuals be accepted by health care plans. For example, the government might mandate that insuring organizations have an open enrollment period in which, anyone must be accepted regardless of health condition. It might also mandate that health insurance cannot be terminated when individuals lose their jobs. The insuring organization, however, could devise a benefits package that is unacceptable to high-risk individuals or provide a lesser quality of care to these individuals in order to get them to disenroll.

A third alternative is to increase the open-enrollment period from the standard one year to a greater number of years. With a greater number of years, it is more difficult for an insuring organization to predict accurately the degree of illness of the population. After all, nearly everyone becomes seriously ill within a long enough period. Therefore, incentives to search for low-risk enrollees are reduced if a plan realizes that individuals will remain in the plan for longer periods of time. Longer enrollment periods, however, will reduce patient options in choice of health plan. There is yet no evidence on the effects of this trade-off in the literature.

A risk adjustment measure is a fourth alternative. The dollar value of a risk adjustment measure can be applied to managed care firms to avoid cream skimming. Greater amounts of money would be paid to insuring organizations that enroll higher risk individuals. If calculated properly, the adjustment creates incentives to enroll high-risk individuals rather than to ignore them. There are a number of potential risk adjusters, no one of which completely accounts for the variance in case mix that managed care firms may have. Indeed, risk adjusters have been criticized by Joseph P. Newhouse ["Patients at Risk: Health Reform and Risk Adjustment," *Health Affairs*, Spring 1994, pp. 132–146], who suggests that it is difficult to devise a risk adjustment measure that captures the predicted variance in expenditures in a given population. For example, Arlene Ash et al. ["Adjusting Medicare Capitation Payments Using Prior Hospitalization Data," *Health Care Financing Review*, Summer 1989, pp. 17–30] used diagnostic cost groups (DCGs) for diseases diagnosed during a prior year's hospitalization. Although this explained a greater amount of the predictable variance, it does not, of course, take into account people who would have substantial outpatient visits, are chronically ill, and have been hospitalized over a period of time [Wynand van de Ven et al., "Risk-Adjusted Capitation: Recent Experiences in the Netherlands," *Health Affairs*, Winter 1994, pp. 120–136].

A sixth alternative may be the use of mandatory high-risk pooling. Each managed care firm would be allowed to place a number of its high-risk enrollees in a pool of all high-risk enrollees. Costs for the high-risk enrollees would be borne by the managed care firms. It is believed that this added safety net would reduce some of the incentives for cream skimming.

Mandatory high-risk pooling would not in itself be able to completely eliminate cream skimming, but it could be viewed as a supplement to a risk-adjustment measure [Erik M. van Barneveld et al., "Mandatory High-Risk Pooling: A Means for Reducing the Incentives for Cream-Skimming," unpublished monograph, Erasmus University, October 3, 1995].

Risk adjustment measures need only be marginally better than the ability of managed care firms to conduct cream skimming. Measures such as standard, uniform benefit packages, absence of preexisting condition exclusion clauses, and open-enrollment periods would also help curtail this behavior, although it is possible that these measures can shift cream skimming in other directions [Katherine Swartz, "Reducing Risk Selection Requires More Than Risk Adjustments," *Inquiry*, 32 (Spring 1995): 6–10].

Managed Care and Its Effects on Competition

Managed care firms compete against fee-for-service plans as well as other managed care firms. Because of the ability of HMOs to achieve lower hospital utilization, they may have a competitive effect on fee-for-service plans. Early evidence has suggested that HMO competition may also make fee-for-service plans adopt utilization review measures to keep people out of the hospital as well. The evidence also showed that fee-for-service plans increase their benefit packages to make them akin to the larger benefit packages of the HMO [Lawrence G. Goldberg and Warren Greenberg, "The Competitive Response of Blue Cross to the Health Maintenance Organization," *Economic Inquiry*, 18 (1980): 57–72].

Roger Feldman and Bryan Dowd found in their study of the state of Minnesota ["The Effectiveness of Managed Competition in Reducing the Costs of Health Insurance," in R. B. Helms, ed., *Health Policy Reform: Competition and Controls* (Washington, DC: American Enterprise Institute for Public Policy Research, 1993), pp. 176–217] that managed competition (not just managed care plans) can have an effect on the costs of the Minnesota group insurance program for state employees. Since Minnesota began offering, in 1989, an array of managed care and fee-for-service plans but paid an amount equal to the cost of the low-cost carrier, 5.9 percent of actual premiums were saved in 1993 as employees enrolled in lower-cost health plans between 1989 and 1993 [p. 212]. These results however, may be due more to the fixed amount paid by the state of Minnesota than to the nature of managed competition plans, since those seeking a more expensive plan have to pay for it entirely with their own funds.

The effect of managed care competitors on costs or premiums of health care firms is complicated by the incentives that insuring organizations have to conduct cream skimming. Roger Feldman et al. found that HMOs raise premiums rather than lower them in their analysis of 239 Minnesota employers in 1986 ["The Effect of HMOs on Premiums in Employment-Based

Health Plans," *Health Services Research*, 27 (1993): 779–811]. Initially, Feldman found higher premiums in HMOs relative to fee-for-service plans because of the more comprehensive coverage of the HMOs. When HMOs competed against fee-for-service plans, the fee-for-service plans lost some of their healthiest patients to HMOs. This increased their costs, and the weighted average of HMO and FFS premiums increased.

Douglas Wholey and colleagues have examined the effects of HMOs on HMO premiums ["The Effect of Market Structure on HMO Premiums," *Journal of Health Economics*, 14 (1995): 81–105]. They find in their pooled time series, cross-sectional analysis that between 1988 and 1991, the greater the number of HMOs, the lower the HMO premiums in a number of market areas in the United States.

As Harold S. Luft suggests ["HMOs, Market Competition, and Premium Cost," *Journal of Health Economics*, 14 (1995): 115–119], the causality of HMO penetration and HMO premiums depends on the assumption that HMOs operate in a reasonably competitive market. That is, there are low entry barriers and some information available to consumers when they make choices among HMOs. It also depends on whether market structural competition is defined by number of firms or a concentration measure. In addition to the structural variables of concentration and number of firms, Wholey et al. used as control measures per capita income and hospital utilization per capita, which may cause shifts in the demand for health care services. Although the authors' results are consistent with economic theory, the analysis is complicated by the potentially high costs of sicker enrollees rather than industrial organization economics only. A more costly case mix should raise premiums, and indeed Wholey and his colleagues found this to be the case for existing HMOs. However, Wholey found that the number of HMOs (rather than market share) can influence fee-for-service plans to reduce premiums, and this in turn results in lower premiums overall for HMOs. It is unclear why the most robust results are with thirteen or more HMOs in a market. This seems like a large number of HMOs needed for a reduction in premiums, especially with such a differentiated product as well as ancillary competition from PPO and POS plans and other types of alternative delivery systems.

Lawrence C. Baker and Kenneth S. Corts, in their analysis of 1,061 employers throughout the United States in 1991, found a new twist in their results ["HMO Penetration and the Cost of Health Care: Market Discipline or Market Segmentation?" *Health Economics*, 86 (1996): 389–394]. They find that at market shares lower than 10 percent, HMOs have a negative effect on the premiums of traditional insurers, but at market shares between 20 and 30 percent, premiums of traditional insurers increased, presumably because of their increasing enrollment of sicker individuals.

Although most studies examine what the effects of HMO competition are at a single point in time, James C. Robinson ["HMO Market Penetration and Hospital Cost Inflation," *Journal of the American Medical Association*,

266 (1991): 2719–2723] examines the effects of the HMO market share for a six-year period between 1982 and 1988. Robinson finds that HMO market penetration in California, calculated as the ratio of HMO-covered hospital admissions to total hospital admissions, had a positive effect on reducing hospital cost increases, defined as the change in the logarithm of hospital costs per admission. These results, however, may understate any competitive effect. It is possible that as HMO competition intensifies, more patients will be treated in out-patient clinics, with only the sickest patients treated on an in-patient basis [p. 2723].

HMOs and Choice of Insuring Organization

Competition among managed care plans should result in lower premiums if consumers compare premiums among managed care plans. The fact that consumers do, indeed, choose among managed care plans is demonstrated by evidence from Dowd and Feldman and Buchmueller and Feldstein. Bryan Dowd and Roger Feldman ["Premium Elasticities of Health Plan Choice," *Inquiry*, 31 (1994–1995): 438–444] found an elasticity of demand of −7.9, based on out-of-pocket premiums, when individuals from five Minnesota employers made health plan choices. The plans covered in their analysis include fee-for-service as well as managed care plans.

Thomas C. Buchmueller and Paul J. Feldstein ["The Effect of Price on Switching Among Health Plans," unpublished monograph, August 1995] found in their examination of University of California health plan offerings that individuals with premium increases below $10.00 switched plans at a rate five times greater than individuals with no premium increases between 1993 and 1994. The authors found that HMO enrollees switch at a faster rate than individuals in fee-for-service plans. This result is not surprising, given the results of the Hellinger study [1995], which showed that individuals who are ill and enrolled in fee-for-service plans are reluctant to switch to managed care plans that limit choice of physician.

System Integration

Before the cost-conscious insuring organization, hospitals and physicians had no incentives to be efficient. Indeed, the more costly providers were, the more they were reimbursed. With the large increase in number and size of managed care firms, however, doctors and hospitals are encouraged to be as efficient as firms in any other industry. Business entities that are not efficient lose customers and decrease their occupancy levels or workload.

It should be pointed out, however, that a simultaneous relationship appears to exist between the demand side (managed care organizations) and the supply side (hospitals and physicians). As Victor R. Fuchs suggests, the "excess" supply of physicians, hospitals, and medical facilities enabled managed care firms to become more cost conscious ["Managed Care and Merger Mania," *Journal of the American Medical Association*, 277 (1997): 920–921]. Moreover, new technology has enabled shifts to less invasive and less costly methods of treating patients.

Firms have attempted to become efficient in a number of ways. On a horizontal level, hospitals have merged in attempts to achieve economies of scale. Efficiencies, for example, may stem from reduced duplication of facilities, fixed costs spread over a greater number of services produced, and economies of buying new assets.

Vertically integrated physician-hospital organizations may be able to achieve some efficiencies with more dependable referral patterns. Physicians who have ties with hospitals can be reasonably assured of a certain level of quality with which they are familiar. Vertical integration may also improve coordination of ambulatory and in-patient visits [Warren Greenberg, "Marshfield Clinic, Physician Networks, and the Exercise of Monopoly Power," draft manuscript, 1998]. Risks in fixed-fee contracts can also be jointly shared between hospitals and physicians. There can be greater coordination of budget policies and clinical practices [Stephen M. Shortell et. al., "The New World of Managed Care: Creating Organized Delivery Systems," *Health Affairs*, Winter 1994, pp. 46–64].

The effects of vertical integration on the performance of the health care sector are unclear. Costs may decline if firms become more efficient. It is possible that access may decrease as less efficient entities are displaced from the market. It is uncertain that quality of care will be affected, although there may be greater coordination of care. Recently, however, there has been a trend toward contractual or virtual integration, although these relationships are not as secure as longer-term vertical relationships. [see James C. Robinson, "Physician-Hospital Integration and the Economic Theory of the Firm," *Medical Care Research and Review*, 54 (1997): 3–24].

Health Insurance and the Uninsured

Approximately 15 percent of the population of the United States does not have health insurance coverage. Aside from equity concerns, individuals are less productive in the marketplace if they are not able to secure medical help [Katherine Swartz, "Dynamics of People Without Health Insurance," *Journal of the American Medical Association*, 271 (1994): 64–66]. Individuals who are hospitalized have a greater chance of dying when they do not have health insurance [Peter Franks et al., "Health and Mortality: Evidence from a National Cohort," *Journal of the American Medical Association* 270 (1993): 737–741]. Women who are not insured have a lesser chance of surviving breast cancer than women who have private insurance [John Z.

Ayanian et al., "The Relation between Health Insurance Coverage and Clinical Outcomes Among Women with Breast Cancer," *New England Journal of Medicine*, 329 (1993): 326–331]. Jack Hadley, Earl Steinberg, and Judith Feder, in their national sample ["Comparison of Uninsured and Privately Insured Hospital Patients," *Journal of the American Medical Association*, 265 (1991): 374–379], found that uninsured patients had a higher chance of dying on admission to a hospital than individuals who were privately insured. Once admitted to the hospital, the uninsured were less likely to have high-discretion procedures.

Chapter 6 shows that, because of the Medicare program, lack of health insurance is not a concern for senior citizens, the severely disabled, and those with kidney disease. The Medicaid program thus far covers individuals under the Aid to Families with Dependent Children provision. The uninsured rate, however, was 17 percent of the nonelderly U.S. population or more than 37 million individuals in 1992 compared to 26.2 million people uninsured or 13.8 percent of the nonelderly population in 1977 [Diane Rowland et al., "A Profile of the Uninsured in America," *Health Affairs*, 11 (1994): 283–287; Lawrence D. Brown, "The Medically Uninsured: Problems, Policies, and Politics," *Journal of Health Politics, Policy, and Law*, 15 (1990): 413–426]. More than 70 percent of the uninsured are not poor and have incomes above the federal poverty level. Indeed, 84 percent of those who are uninsured have full-time or part-time jobs or are dependents of those who have jobs [Rowland et al., pp. 284–285]. Moreover, even some individuals who have health insurance may have preexisting medical conditions under which preexisting condition clauses may preclude treatment payment.

In addition to the uninsured, there are individuals who are underinsured. Thomas Bodenheimer describes the underinsured as those with "large" out-of-pocket payments ["Underinsurance in America," *New Enland Journal of Medicine*, 327 (1992): 274–278]. This may add another 20 million people to the roster without adequate coverage [p. 274], although large out-of-pocket expenses may put a brake on health care costs and may be a goal of those who favor catastrophic insurance.

The literature has recently pointed out, however, that the uncertainty of not having health insurance during a period of time compared to a single point in time is not insignificant. In a 1993 survey, Karen Davis et al. found that one-third of adults had been uninsured at some point during the previous two years of their survey ["Health Insurance: The Size and Shape of the Problem," *Inquiry*, 32 (1995): 196–203]. Katherine Swartz estimated that the total number of individuals insured at some time during 1992 was 58 million people ["Dynamics of People Without Health Insurance," *Journal of the American Medical Association*, 271 (1994): 64–66]. Swartz and Timothy D. McBride found that, using a 1984 data set, 15 percent of all uninsured spells are greater than 24 months in length ["Spells Without Health Insurance: Distributions of Durations and Their Link to Point-in-Time Estimates of the Uninsured," *Inquiry*, 27 (1990): 281–288].

Health Care Marketplace

Ocean State Physicians Health Plan, Inc., et al. v. *Blue Cross and Blue Shield of Rhode Island* (1988) confronts a number of antitrust issues from the demand side as well as from the perspective of the overall health care marketplace. Blue Cross and Blue Shield was, by a large market share margin, the dominant health insurer in Rhode Island, with more than 75 percent of insured people from at least the early 1970s to the initiation of the complaint. (Blue Cross and Blue Shield were separate plans, each with more than 70 percent of the market, until they merged in 1982.) The BC/BS exemption from various property and premium taxes because of their non-profit status created barriers to entry for new for-profit insurers and managed care plans. In addition, Blue Cross and Blue Shield received a 13 percent discount on hospital charges, which enabled them to realize lower costs [Goldberg and Greenberg, 1995].

Since the mid-1980's, however, the enrollment in alternative delivery systems in Rhode Island has increased rapidly. Ocean State's health plan had grown from 565 members in 1983 to approximately 123,864 members in 1990. Ocean State had been the fastest-growing HMO, although the combined enrollment of the four alternative delivery systems that remained in the market was more than 222,000 in 1990 [Goldberg and Greenberg, p. 67].

In 1986, Blue Cross and Blue Shield responded to the growth of Ocean State in three distinct ways. First, it responded with the introduction of a most-favored nation (MFN) clause, which stated that Ocean State would not pay physicians higher fees than other insurers were paying. Second, Blue Cross and Blue Shield offered a preferred provider organization (PPO), HealthMate, which was similar to Ocean State in its restricted choice of physicians but had more comprehensive benefits than traditional Blue Cross and Blue Shield.

The third response was to institute an adverse selection policy. Under this policy, Blue Cross and Blue Shield would charge their highest premium to employers if they offered to their employees Ocean State Physicians Health Plan and traditional Blue Cross and Blue Shield. If Ocean State were offered, Blue Cross and Blue Shield was concerned that employees who were in poorer health would select the Blue Cross and Blue Shield plan, which would increase their premiums relative to the Ocean State HMO. A lower premium would be charged to induce the employer to also offer Health Mate to capture some of the purported good risks from Ocean State. Finally, the employer would receive the lowest premium if traditional Blue Cross and Blue Shield were alone offered to the employee. In this case, of course, there could be no adverse selection.

The Blue Cross and Blue Shield offering of HealthMate and the reduction in price for HealthMate to employers who offered all three plans appeared to be noncontroversial. Blue Cross and Blue Shields actions appeared to be legitimate competitive responses to a new entrant. The implementation of the MFN clause, however, carried a number of costs and benefits. Blue Cross and Blue Shield may be viewed as attempting to achieve the lowest price possible for physician services and was, therefore, acting as a cost-conscious insurer, driving down the price of physician services. Ocean State, however, asserted in its complaint against Blue Cross and Blue Shield that it would not be able to recruit physicians into its plan because physicians would reject its attempts to pay lower fees because they would also have to accept a lower fee from Blue Cross and Blue Shield. Ocean State asserted that because of the MFN it would have a harder time attracting physicians and remaining in the marketplace. Nevertheless, through utilization review or other financial incentives, there were many other ways for Ocean State to contain costs and be competitive. Indeed, as we have seen, Ocean State experienced high growth rates despite the existence of Blue Cross and Blue Shield's MFN clause. The U.S. District Court ruled in favor of Blue Cross and Blue Shield and was affirmed by the U.S. Court of Appeals.

Chapter 4 Appendix

Ocean State Physicians Health Plan, Inc., et al., Plaintiffs, Appellants,
v.
Blue Cross & Blue Shield of Rhode Island, Defendant, Appellee

No. 88-1851
U.S. Court of Appeals,
First Circuit
Decided August 21, 1989

Blue Cross initiated a policy, which it called "Prudent Buyer," of not paying a physician more for any service or procedure than that physician was accepting from any other health care cost provider (such as Ocean State). Blue Cross established this policy after it became apparent that Ocean State's contracting physicians were accepting about 20 percent less for their services from Ocean State than they were receiving from Blue Cross. Ocean State had withheld 20 percent of its physicians' fees in 1985, with the expectation that if the corporation made a profit the withhold would be returned. Ocean State did not turn a profit, however, and the withhold was not returned. In 1986 Ocean State again withheld 20 percent of its physician fees, which it again failed to return after the end of the year. In order to ensure that it was getting the physicians' best prices, Blue Cross required each of its participating physicians to certify that he or she was not accepting any lower fees from other providers than he or she was receiving from Blue Cross for the same service. If the provider failed to provide such certification, Blue Cross reduced that physician's fees by 20 percent. As a result of the Prudent Buyer policy, Blue Cross achieved significant cost savings. After the implementation of Prudent Buyer, about 350 of Ocean State's 1200 physicians resigned, in many cases apparently in order to avoid a reduction in their Blue Cross fees (pp. 1103–1104).

The Prudent Buyer policy involves Blue Cross's relationships not with its subscribers but with its provider physicians.... We agree with the district court, however, that the Prudent Buyer policy—through which Blue Cross ensured that it would not pay a provider physician any more for any particular service than she was accepting from Ocean State or any other private health care purchaser—is, as a matter of law, not violative of section 2 of the Sherman Act....

In the case at hand, the record amply supports Blue Cross's view that Prudent Buyer was a bona fide policy to ensure that Blue Cross would not pay more than any competitor paid for the same services. According to the policy, when physicians provided data on the lowest prices they accepted for particular services, and these prices were lower than those allowed by Blue Cross, Blue Cross lowered its price to match the lowest price accepted. When Ocean State physicians did not provide this price information, Blue Cross reduced its fee to the physicians by 20%, to correspond to Ocean State's 20% withhold. Blue Cross estimated that it saved $1,900,000 through this policy.

We agree with the district court that such a policy of insisting on a supplier's lowest price—assuming that the price is not "predatory" or below the supplier's incremental cost—tends to further competition on the merits and, as a matter of law, is not exclusionary. It is hard to disagree with the district court's view:

As a naked proposition, it would seem silly to argue that a policy to pay the same amount for the same service is anticompetitive, even on the part of one who has market power. This, it would seem, is what competition should be all about (p. 1110).

5
Employer and Employee as Purchasers of Health Care Services

More than 90 percent of nonelderly individuals who have health insurance in the private sector in the United States receive their coverage from their employer ["Trends in Health Insurance Coverage," *EBRI Issue Brief 185*, May 1997, Table 1, p. 5]. Employer-sponsored health insurance, however, is not essential for the distribution of health insurance. Residents of Canada, Israel, and the Netherlands, for example, do not receive health care coverage from their employer (Chapter 11).

Employer-based health insurance in the United States became much more common after the imposition of wage and price controls during World War II. To increase compensation in order to compete for prospective employees, employers began to offer payment of health insurance premiums. The employer-based health insurance system in the private sector in the United States imposes costs on the U.S. economy, especially in terms of mobility of resources, equity of coverage, and efficiency in health care and labor markets.

The incentives of the employer are to contain health care costs and to offer plans with good quality medical care in an effort to attract the best possible employees and contribute to maximizing the profits of the firm. The employer also has incentives to minimize transactions costs in its offering of health care plans. Each plan offered means additional costs of negotiating terms and premiums. Furthermore, a large array of plans can mean that each plan has to spread risk over a fewer number of employees, which can result in a higher risk premium for each plan.

Costs of Employer-Based Health Insurance

The incentives of the employee are to enroll in the best quality health care plan at the lowest possible cost. The incentives, however, of the employer and the employee may diverge, and the incentives of both may diverge from the interests of society as a whole. For example, premiums paid by the employer are tax-deductible expenses for the firm and they are excluded from the taxable income of employees. No Social Security, Medicare, or income taxes are applied toward these premiums. Thus, the employer has an incentive to provide more health insurance than would be the case if premiums were taxed in the same way as income. Employees have incentives to demand more health insurance for the same reason, disproportionately benefiting those in the higher tax brackets. Because of the tax incentives, employers pay approximately 80 percent of health care premiums, on average, and employees pay the remainder [Peter Budetti, "Universal Health Care Coverage—Pitfalls and Promise of an Employment-Based Approach," *Journal of Medicine and Philosophy*, 17 (1992): pp. 21–32, p. 22]. Excess health insurance leads to greater quantities of health services bought at higher prices. Martin S. Feldstein has suggested that there is a significant welfare loss (or loss to society of too many resources consumed) ["The Welfare Loss of Excess Health Insurance," *Journal of Political Economy*, March–April 1973, pp. 251–279].

According to a 1991 Health Insurance Association of America survey, 40 percent of firms did not offer health insurance to employees [Cynthia B. Sullivan et al., "Employer-Sponsored Health Insurance in 1991," *Health Affairs*, Winter 1992, pp. 172–185]. Only 42 percent of medium- and large-size firms offered a choice of health insurance plans. Among smaller firms, only 6 percent offered a choice of health plans ["Choice of Health Plans Among Full-Time Workers," *EBRI Notes*, 17 (August 1996): 2].

Lack of choice may stem from the transactions costs of selecting and offering more than one plan or the presence of a limited number of health plans in an area. Employers might also not want to duplicate HMO coverage. Choice, however, could improve consumer welfare as well as stimulate competition among plans based on price and quality.

There is evidence that lower-income workers over time are less likely to have employer-based health insurance coverage. Richard Kronick ["Health Insurance, 1979–1989: The Frayed Connection Between Employment and Insurance," *Inquiry*, 28 (Winter 1991): 318–332] found more than a 10 percent decline in employer-based coverage of workers earning $6.00 per hour in 1989 compared to 1979.

Employers may choose not to offer health insurance because of cost. The average cost in 1994 was $3,420 per employee ["Portability of Health Insurance: COBRA Expansions and Small Group Market Reform," *EBRI Issue Brief 166*, October 1995, p. 1]. Transactions costs can be substantial for firms that continually register new employees for health care benefits in high-turnover industries such as real estate, automotive repairs, and building construction. Currently, there are approximately 27 million individuals employed in these industries, according to Alvin L. Schorr ["Job Turnover—A Problem with Employer-Based Health Care," *New England Journal of Medicine*, 323 (1990): 543–545], although the exact definition of a high-turnover industry is unclear. In addition, of course, all industries have some turnover.

Transactions costs may also explain why larger firms are more apt to offer health insurance coverage than smaller firms. In the private sector, 33 percent of workers in companies with fewer than ten employees were uninsured, compared with 11.6 percent of workers in private sector firms with 1,000 or more employees ["Sources of Health Insurance and Characteristics of the Uninsured, Analysis of the March 1996 Current Population Survey," *EBRI Issue Brief 179*, November 1996, p. 17]. Peter Diamond ["Organizing the Health Insurance Market," *Econometrica*, 60 (1992): 1233–1254] has compiled estimates from the Congressional Budget Office and the Hay-Higgins Company that for groups from one to four, the ratio of administrative costs to benefit costs is 40 percent for the insuring organization, while for groups of 10,000 or more the ratio is 5.5 percent. The Employee Benefit Research Institute, from its analysis of Current Population Survey data, shows that the greater the size of a firm, the more likely it is to offer health insurance. ["Sources of Health Insurance and Characteristics of the Uninsured," *EBRI Issue Brief 123* March 1991, Table 25, p. 52]. Of course, firms with a greater number of employees can more easily spread the risks of a few high-cost individuals.

Job Lock and Employer-Provided Health Insurance

Approximately 15 percent of the adult work force retain their current jobs because of the possibility of not being able to secure health care benefits on a subsequent job—the so-called job lock phenomenon [International Communications Research Survey Research Group, Excel Omnibus Study, December 7–11, 1990, Table 4, p. 4]. Individuals who want to return to school, to work part time, or to begin their own firm, continue in unproductive jobs because they would not be able to afford health insurance or would have sharply reduced health benefits without their current job. Health care benefits may be difficult to obtain from a new employer because, for example, a family member might have a preexisting condition. Many potential employers do not provide any health insurance to employees. There have been no studies of estimates of the loss of productivity to society for those who cannot change jobs or who have switched jobs because of health care benefits. There were approximately 125 million employed civilians in the United States work force in 1995 with an average wage or salary of approximately $27,000 a year [U.S. Department of Commerce, *Statistical Abstract of the United States, 1995*, Table 615, p. 393, and Table 661, p. 425]. Assume that forced retention or job change resulted in a productivity loss of just 5 percent of income, or $1,350 per worker. Fifteen percent of 125 million workers (18.75 million) multiplied by $1,350 is equal to a $25.3 billion productivity loss in a single year. This loss, of course, varies depending on the probability of obtaining a job with health insurance benefits and the actual size of the productivity loss. Philip F. Cooper and Alan C. Monheit ["Does Employment-Related Health Insurance Inhibit Job Mobility?"

Inquiry 30 (1993): 400–416], using 1987 National Medical Expenditure Survey data in their multivariate analysis, also found that the presence of health insurance benefits on the job deterred individuals from switching jobs for fear of losing health insurance.

Under the Consolidated Omnibus Budget Reconciliation Act of 1985 (COBRA), employees and their dependents (in firms with twenty or more employees) who have group health insurance can maintain their coverage after they leave a firm. COBRA has not been a satisfactory bridge to full coverage, however, because premiums for the continuation coverage cost up to 102 percent of the total premium of the plan and COBRA coverage generally terminates within eighteen months ["Portability of Health Insurance: COBRA Expansions and Small Group Market Reform," *EBRI Issue Brief 166*, October 1995, pp. 1–5].

The Health Insurance Portability and Accountability Act (the Kassebaum-Kennedy bill), passed in 1996, does little to alleviate many of the problems of employer-based health insurance. The Act primarily helps individuals with preexisting conditions who would like to move from one firm to another but retain a health insurance benefit. If individuals were employed in their former firm for more than 12 months, they are immediately eligible for health care coverage in their new firm regardless of any preexisting conditions. The waiting period is increased for preexisting conditions by one month for every month fewer than twelve that one had insurance at the former job. The health care plans offered, however, may be different in the second firm compared to the first. The Kassebaum-Kennedy bill will also raise costs to firms that provide health insurance because of the potential risk and cost of insuring high-cost workers. Individuals who wish to join a firm that does not offer health insurance or who wish to begin their own business can buy health insurance on an individual basis with no preexisting condition exceptions if they worked for their previous employer for twelve months or more. However, insuring organizations may charge premiums based on the health condition and preexisting condition status of the person, putting health insurance out of reach for many people in poor health.

"Reverse" job lock might be experienced by firms that offer extensive health care benefits. Individuals who have little or no health benefits might, after becoming ill, take jobs in firms that offer more complete benefits, increasing costs for the new employer. Incentives will grow for the new employer to reduce or eliminate coverage for new employees to avoid increased health care costs through adverse selection. This can further exacerbate the problem of immobility and job lock and can increase the number of uninsured. Further, individuals who receive Medicaid payments may be reluctant to seek employment in industries that ordinarily do not offer health insurance for fear of losing their Medicaid coverage [Paul Starr, *The Logic of Health-Care Reform* (Knoxville, TN: Grand Rounds Press, 1992), p. 23], thus further reducing the productivity of the work force.

Additional Costs of Employer-Based Health Insurance

Individuals who have lost their jobs because of a company's bankruptcy can also lose their health insurance ["Retirees' Plight in Bankruptcies," *New York Times*, July 2, 1991, p. D1]. Similarly, individuals who have been employed by those firms and are now retired may lose retiree health benefits. Approximately 13 million people over the age of 55 are retired and receive such benefits, which are especially important before becoming eligible for Medicare ["Retirees Threatened with Loss of Insurance," *New York Times*, June 28, 1992, p. 1]. In a recession, of course, firms have additional incentives to reduce health care benefits.

Individuals who currently have health care coverage with their employer through self-insured plans may also be at risk for loss of this coverage. In the U.S. Court of Appeals decision, *McGann* v. *H&H Music Company, et al.* (946 F. d 401, November 4, 1991), the opinion of the United States District Court for the Southern District of Texas allowed H&H Music Company to drastically reduce insurance coverage for John McGann, who was infected with the AIDS virus (see Appendix). Previously, the policy would have paid up to $1 million in health care costs for AIDS for the lifetime of an employee. After the reduction, the company could choose to pay only $5,000 for the lifetime cost of AIDS. The courts ruled that reductions in health benefits were permissible for firms that were self-insured. These firms are exempt from state insurance regulations and subject only to the Employee Retirement Income Security Act (ERISA) provisions, which do not mandate the size and scope of benefit packages. Reductions can take place without warning to the employee. In November 1992, the Supreme Court refused to consider the case further, thereby letting the lower court decision stand ["Justices Leave Intact Ruling That Lets Business Cut Health Benefits," *New York Times*, November 10, 1992, p. A18]. According to the courts, the reduction in health insurance benefits by a self-insured firm is not much different than reduction in any other fringe benefits, such as vacation benefits. Firms are free to provide or not to provide benefits depending on their financial position or their competitive positions in attracting employees.

The H&H decision may increase the amount of uncertainty among employees of self-insured firms (and the extent to which individuals even know that they are employed by self-insured firms is not clear) about the amount of health care expenses that they themselves may have to incur in the future. The decision also removed most state regulation of self-insured health care plans. The decision, however, allowed employers to be more flexible in containing the total labor costs of the firm.

Employer-based health care imposes other limitations on access to health insurance coverage. Individuals who are not in the labor force generally cannot secure this kind of coverage. Health insurance firms avoid individuals who are not in the labor force because these individuals are generally in poorer health than the remainder of the population [Donald W. Light, "The Practice and Ethics of Risk-Related Health Insurance," *Journal of the American Medical Association*, 257 (1992): 2503–2508]. Under the Americans with Disabilities Act of 1990 (P. L. 101–336, 104 Stat. 327), prospective job applicants may not be asked their health status prior to employment. Since, by law, workers with disabilities now must receive the same health care coverage as the rest of the work force, employers have incentives to reduce health coverage or request high copayments from all workers. As more individuals with disabilities are employed, employers will have greater incentives to reduce health care coverage for all or to eliminate health care coverage entirely ["Disabilities Law Could Have a Big Impact on Health Care Benefits," *Washington Post*, January 3, 1993, p. H2].

Employers may not be able to offer a health insurance plan to high-risk employees. Groups of gay activists or individuals who work with asbestos, for example, have had difficulty in securing coverage from *any* insurance firm [Light, 1992]. Furthermore, since a large number of small firms is experienced rated, the result is potentially wide-ranging differences in premiums for different groups. Small groups may be sensitive to this since the premiums of a few individuals with disabilities in a group may raise premiums considerably [Katherine Swartz, "Why Requiring Employers to Provide Health Insurance is a Bad Idea," *Journal of Health Politics, Policy and Law*, 15 (1990): 779–792].

Even if individuals are offered health insurance by their employer, adverse selection may occur. With no risk adjustment, individuals with high-cost illnesses will most likely select the more comprehensive plans, driving up the costs of these plans. A risk adjustment is needed here as it is needed in any setting where there is competition among health insuring organizations. One can see this most clearly with the Federal Employees Health Benefits Program (FEHBP), a plan established in 1959 for federal retirees and active workers. Under the FEHBP all federal workers can choose from at least twenty different plans [Marlilyn J. Field and Harold T. Shapiro, eds. *Employment and Health Benefits* (Washington, DC: National Academy Press, 1993)], including fee-for-service and managed care plans. The Field and Shapiro report notes that the FEHBP program suffers from "serious" adverse risk selection problems [p. 175]. Although the federal government partially mitigates the adverse selection problem by paying 60 percent of the premiums of the average of the most expensive six plans (not to exceed a 75 percent contribution to any single plan), cream skimming occurred [p. 73].

Individuals who remain with the same employer might generate higher costs if the employer decides to offer a different menu of insuring organizations. Individuals have to select a new insuring organization, which might involve a new series of duplicate tests and visits from a different group of physicians. Individuals who change employers might be subject to a new set of insuring organizations, which might also mean duplicate tests and visits.

The current employer-based system includes individuals who have coverage from their own employer and from their spouse's employer. This can result in increased transactions costs for both the employee and the two insuring organizations in order to coordinate benefits between the two plans. According to data of the Employee Benefit Research Institute, 10 percent of individuals had more than one source of group health coverage in 1991 ["Sources of Health Insurance and Characteristics of the Uninsured, Analysis of the March 1991 Current Population Survey," *EBRI Special Report and Issue Brief 123*, February 1992].

Another possible cost of the employer-based system is the increased use of Medicaid benefits instead of employer-sponsored insurance by those who have recently become eligible for Medicaid under its recently expanded provisions. The inadequacy and uncertainty of dependable private sector employer-based benefits may be another reason why individuals select Medicaid benefits, although Medicaid is known for its lack of physician participation, its poor service in some areas, and its lack of convenience. In their analysis, David M. Cutler and Jonathan Gruber ["The Effect of Medicaid Expansions on Public Insurance, Private Insurance, and Redistribution," *American Economic Review*, 86 (1996): 378–383] suggest that the increase in Medicaid eligibility is crowding out private health insurance, with higher costs for the Medicaid program. Cutler and Gruber report that Medicaid coverage increased by 2.2 million enrollees between 1987 and 1992, while private sector coverage declined by 1.7 million during this period.

What are the advantages of the current employer-based system? Employers may be able to provide information on the costs and benefits of various plans at lower costs than if individuals were to purchase plans without regard to employer attachment. The corporate coalitions may be able to secure more data on characteristics of providers in the coalition. If these data improve outcomes, however, the data may have benefits external to members of the coalition and should be available to all. The employer-based system may also have the advantage of being able to pool individuals with diverse risks into a single group. But even though risks in a group are pooled, there may still be large differences in premiums and risks among the different health care plans that are offered.

Can Employers Achieve Lower Health Care Costs?

Employers are analogous to car rental firms like Hertz or Avis, which buy automobiles from automobile manufacturers at lower prices than individuals would pay. The average price of all cars sold does not go down or quality increase because there is a large buyer in the marketplace. It is the same in health care. Employees of the large firm may achieve lower prices, but costs may increase for others. Some savings may be generated by a reduction in transactions costs or economies of scale in large purchases. Also, the pooling of risks helps higher-risk individuals. Thus, any single employee may enjoy some cost savings from joining an employer group, but little significant savings may accrue to society as a whole.[1]

In many geographic areas, a number of employers have joined together to form health care coalitions. These coalitions attempt to contain health care costs and to ensure high-quality health care for their employees. But what can health care coalitions do that individual employer firms cannot? They may exert some monopsonistic power. If health insuring organizations have competitive rates of return, however, it would be difficult to achieve lower prices from them on an aggregate basis. Chapter 4 has already shown that there are no barriers to entry in the health insuring market that would deter new firms from bidding away excess profits. It is also not clear how a group of firms would be able to achieve greater increases in quality of care. Each health insuring organization or each employer that buys from a health insuring organization has its own incentives to achieve the quality of care it desires. Health care coalitions may, however, be effective in collecting more information on provider costs and quality in order to help improve performance.

Health Care Marketplace

The legal case in the Appendix illustrates a potential uncertainty of retaining health insurance when one is employed with a medium or small-sized, self-insured firm. Although most self-insured firms are larger firms with strong unions, the H&H Music Company, a medium-sized firm, was allowed to terminate the health insurance of an employee, with less than twenty-four hours notice.

---

[1] Jack A. Meyer [August 1997] has made the point to me that large employers or managed care firms may change the practice patterns of providers in the community, resulting in cost savings.

Chapter 5 Appendix

John McGann, Plaintiff-Appellant,
v.
H&H MUSIC COMPANY, et al.,
Defendants-Appellees
No. 90-2672

United States Court of Appeals,
Fifth Circuit
Decided November 4, 1991

McGann, an employee of H&H Music, discovered that he was afflicted with AIDS in December 1987. Soon thereafter, McGann submitted his first claim for reimbursement under H&H Music's group medical plan, provided through Brook Mays, the plan administrator, and issued by General American, the plan insurer, and informed his employer that he had AIDS. McGann met with officials of H&H Music in March 1988 at which time they discussed McGann's illness. Before the change in the terms of the plan, it provided for lifetime medical benefits of up to $1,000,000 to all employees (p. 403).

In July 1988, H&H Music informed its employees that, effective August 1, 1988, changes would be made in their medical coverage. These changes included, but were not limited to, limitation of benefits payable for AIDS-related claims to a lifetime maximum of $5,000. No limitation was placed on any other catastrophic illness. H&H Music became self-insured under the new plan and General American became the plan's administrator. By January 1990, McGann had exhausted the $5,000 limit on coverage for his illness (p. 403).

In August 1989, McGann sued H&H Music, Brook Mays and General American under Section 510 of ERISA, which provides, in part, as follows:

It shall be unlawful for any person to discharge, fine, suspend, expel, discipline, or discriminate against a participant or beneficiary for exercising any right to which he is entitled under the provisions of an employee benefit plan, or for the purpose of interfering with the attainment of any right to which such participant may become entitled under the plan [29 U.S.C. § 1140] (p. 403)].

Defendants, conced[ed] the factual allegations of McGann's complaint. ... These factual allegations include no assertion that the reduction of AIDS benefits was intended to deny benefits to McGann for any reason which would not be applicable to other beneficiaries who might then or thereafter have AIDS, but rather that the reduction was prompted by the knowledge of McGann's illness, and that McGann was the only beneficiary then known to have AIDS (pp. 403–404).

Although we assume there was a connection between the benefits reduction and either McGann's filing of claims or his revelations about his illness, there is nothing in the record to suggest that defendants' motivation was other than as they asserted, namely to avoid the expense of paying for AIDS treatment (if not, indeed, also for other treatment), no more for McGann than for any other present or future plan beneficiary who might suffer from AIDS. McGann concedes that the reduction in AIDS benefits will apply equally to all employees filing AIDS-related claims and that the effect of the reduction will not necessarily be felt only by him (p. 404).

McGann's allegations show no *promised* benefit, for there is nothing to indicate that defendants ever promised that the $1,000,000 coverage limit was permanent (p. 405).

McGann's claim cannot be reconciled with the well-settled principle that Congress did not intend that ERISA circumscribe employers' control over the content of benefits plans they offered to their employees (p. 407).

Under McGann's theory, defendants would be effectively proscribed from reducing coverage for AIDS once McGann had contracted that illness and filed claims for AIDS-related expenses. If a federal court could prevent an employer from reducing an employee's coverage limits for AIDS treatment once that employee contracted AIDS, the boundaries of judicial involvement in the creation, alteration or termination of ERISA plans would be sorely tested (p. 408).

ERISA does not broadly prevent an employer from "discriminating" in the creation, alteration or termination of employee benefits plans; thus, evidence of such intentional discrimination cannot alone sustain a claim under section 510 (p. 408).

It does not prohibit an employer from electing not to cover or continue to cover AIDS, while covering or continuing to cover other catastrophic illnesses, even though the employer's decision in this respect may stem from some "prejudice" against AIDS or its victims generally. The same, of course, is true of any other disease and its victims (p. 408).

This ruling was left standing by the U.S. Supreme Court. *McGann* v. *H&H Music Co.*, (*cert.denied sub nom* Frank Greenberg, Independent Executor of Estate of John W. McGann, Deceased, Petitioner, v. H&H Music Company, et al., 113 S. Ct. 482, 1992).

6
Health Insurance in the Public Sector

Among other programs, health insurance in the public sector consists primarily of the Medicare program for the elderly, for those on end-stage renal dialysis, and for those who have been disabled for more than twenty-four months. It also consists of the Medicaid program for those who receive Aid to Families with Dependent Children (AFDC) benefits and the provisions of the Supplemental Security Income (SSI) program, which provides cash payments for the aged, blind, and the disabled. Individuals who are "medically needy" because they have used their assets and income for medical expenses are also eligible for Medicaid assistance if they fit into the AFDC and SSI categories.

Another public program, the Veterans Administration (VA), runs the largest centrally directed hospital and clinic system in the United States. The four overlapping groups of veterans eligible to receive benefits are (1) veterans with service-connected disabilities or certain other service-connected qualifying characteristics, such as having been exposed to herbicides in Vietnam; (2) recipients of VA pensions; (3) veterans 65 and older; and (4) veterans meeting certain income means tests [Steven Jonas, *An Introduction to the U.S. Health Care System*, 3rd ed. (New York: Springer Publishing Company, 1992), p. 96]. Expenditures for VA hospitals and medical care were nearly $14.3 billion in 1993 [U.S. Department of Commerce, *Statistical Abstract of the United States 1995*, Table 151. p. 110].

Why are there public health insurance programs when there are private sector programs? The Medicare and Medicaid programs fill the need created by the unwillingness of the private sector to insure potentially high-cost elderly people, people with long-term disabilities, and people who cannot afford to pay for health insurance. The motivating economic factor behind the health insurance programs in the public sector seems to be to provide health insurance coverage to those who may not be able to afford it on their own. The existence of other public programs, such as the VA program, may stem from the special health needs of their client populations.

Public health insurance programs do not mean that the government is necessarily the payor of health care services, nor do they mean that the government necessarily provides health care services. Under the Medicare and Medicaid programs in the United States, the government (or a contractual representative) is almost always the payor of health care services, but it has not served as the provider of health services. When government is the sole payor for health care services the possibility of price competition among providers is often eliminated, and prices set by the government are usually set inefficiently. Since 1982, however, in some Medicaid demonstration programs, price competition among providers has been introduced in a vigorous manner.

The increase in health care costs and its effects on federal and state budgets may have led the governments to search for alternatives; at the same time, rising costs have made it more feasible for managed care systems to enter the marketplace for government beneficiaries. Government may also have realized that health care services can be purchased like other goods and services, as long as government is cognizant about the distribution of the services. At the same time, government-set prices in health care appear to be a prescription for inefficiency in health care. The movement toward a marketplace in health care that encompasses managed care systems appears to be the trend not only in the public and private sectors in the United States but in many countries outside the United States as well.

Medicare

Medicare, or Title XVIII of the Social Security Act, was enacted by the Congress in 1965. The enrollment and expenditures for Medicare between 1966 and 1995, for selected years, are shown in Table 6-1. Enrollment has almost doubled from 19.1 million in 1966 to 37.3 million in 1995. Medicare expenditures have grown more than 100-fold from $1.7 billion in 1966 to nearly $184.0 billion in 1995 [Sources are Table 6-1 next page]. In 1995, Medicare expenditures were 20.9 percent of total national health care expenditures compared with only 4.0 percent in 1966. [U.S. Department of Commerce, *Statistical Abstract of the United States 1968*, p. 63; Katharine R. Levit et al., "National Health Expenditures, 1995," *Health Care Financing Review*, 18 (Fall 1996): Table 1, p. 179; see, also, sources Table 6-1].

Medicare has a standardized benefit package for its beneficiaries in its traditional fee-for-service program. Part A, which is mandatory for all beneficiaries, includes most hospitalizations, out-patient care, such as home care, auxiliary tests performed in the hospital, and hospice services. Skilled nursing facilities (SNF) are covered under Part A if the patient has been hospitalized for at least 3 days within the previous 30 days and is medically necessary [*Health Care Financing Review*, Medicare and Medicaid Supplement (February 1995), p. 4]. Part B, which need not be purchased, pays for most physician and support services as well as ambulance services, medical equipment, and prosthetic devices. In 1996, more than 90 percent of the Medicare population, however, paid $42.50 a month for Part B ["Political

[Handwritten annotations: "Medicare Title XVIII of Soc. Sec. Act, 1965", "SNFs", "1.45%", "2.9%"]

TABLE 6-1. Total Medicare spending and enrollment, selected years 1966–1995

Fiscal years/Calendar years	Medicare Spending (in billions of dollars)	Enrollment (in millions)
1966	1.7	19.1
1967	4.7	19.5
1970	7.2	20.4
1975	16.3	24.9
1980	36.4	28.4
1983	58.0	29.9
1985	70.1	31.0
1990	109.0	34.1
1993	148.4	36.2
1995	183.8	37.3

Source for calendar years 1966–1967: *Health Care Financing Review*, 17 (1996): Table 6, p. 225. Source for calendar years 1970–1980: *Health Care Financing Review*, Medicare and Medicaid Supplement, February 1995, Table 2, p. 152, and Table 5, p. 155. Source for fiscal years 1983–1995: Prospective Payment Assessment Commission, *Medicare and the American Health Care System*, Report to the Congress, June 1996, Table A-1, p. 117, and Table A-2, p. 118.

Stakes Increase in Fight to Save Medicare," *New York Times*, June 3, 1996, p. B-10]. Three-fourths of the costs of Medicare Part B are subsidized from the U.S. Treasury's general operating fund.

Financing of Medicare

Medicare is financed by a mandatory payroll tax on working individuals, similar to the payroll tax that finances the Social Security Trust Fund, which is deposited into Part A, Medicare Trust Fund. Currently, the Medicare tax is 1.45 percent of taxable earnings for employees as well as a 1.45 percent tax on employers. Self-employed individuals pay a 2.9 percent tax [Katharine R. Levit et al., "National Health Expenditures, 1994," *Health Care Financing Review*, 17 (1996), 205–242]. Individuals with supplemental coverage also pay copayments of 20 percent of a physician's Medicare-approved fee[1] if the physician is a participating Medicare physician. A nonparticipating physician may charge the patient up to 15 percent more than the approved fee. Patients must also pay 20 percent of approved amounts for ambulance, medical equipment, and portable devices.

Patients pay an initial deductible equal to the cost of one inpatient day in the hospital for each hospital stay and pay a percentage of the deductible for longer hospital stays. After a sixty-day stay, Medicare requires a payment of one-quarter of the deductible per day until the ninetieth day. After the ninetieth day, Medicare allows each beneficiary only a sixty-day lifetime reserve under which Medicare requires a payment of one-half of the

---

[1] The approved fee is developed under the RBRVS system; see Chapter 2.

deductible per day. After 150 days, the beneficiary is required to pay the hospital's full charge each day. When the lifetime reserve days are used. Medicare coverage ends after a ninety-day length of stay [*Health Care Financing Review*, Medicare and Medicaid Statistical Supplement (February 1995), p. 5]. Contrary to fundamental insurance principles, therefore, Medicare does not provide catastrophic coverage. During the later stages of an illness, when patients most need hospital insurance, Medicare pays a smaller and smaller share of the hospital bill.

In order to cover the medical expenses that Medicare does not pay, 75 percent of beneficiaries [Peter D. Fox et al., "Medigap Regulation: Lessons for Health Care Reform," *Journal of Health Politics, Policy and Law*, 20 (1995): 31–48] purchase "Medigap" insurance coverage, in part to cover the copayments and deductibles. This insurance is contrary to Medicare's goals of cost containment because copayments and deductibles are intended to curtail insurance utilization. Fox et al., however, point out that Medicare pays just 45 percent of health care expenditures incurred by those over 65 [p. 32], which apparently has created a demand for Medigap coverage. Since 1992, the number of Medigap policies has been reduced to a maximum of ten different types in order to reduce the costs of search when individuals decide among many policies. All policies cover the coinsurance and deductibles of Parts A and B, but only three out of ten cover prescription drugs [p. 35]. Premiums may vary among the policies and may reflect the age of the beneficiary. Nevertheless, there may be competition among insurers to avoid potentially high-cost enrollees [p. 46].

Individuals are entitled to Medicare coverage regardless of their prior or current income. Thus, the government provides benefits to all Medicare-eligible individuals over age 65, even though 4.6 percent of them had incomes greater than $75,000 in 1994 [U.S. Department of Commerce, *Statistical Abstract of the United States 1995*, no. 725, p. 470]. Although high-income individuals have also paid taxes, it need not follow that they should be entitled to receive benefits. It is not uncommon for people to pay taxes for government programs but not receive benefits. For example, many people pay for the upkeep of national parks, but not everyone is in a position to enjoy them.

Medicare and Cost-Conscious Behavior

Beginning with the enactment of Medicare in 1965, the federal government paid hospitals on a cost-plus basis and physicians on a reasonable-cost basis, providing little incentive for cost containment by providers. Indeed, a cost-plus basis created perverse incentives: the more inefficient the hospital, the more the hospital was paid. A reasonable-cost basis for physicians allowed physicians to continually bill higher fees. These payment schemes were not unlike the cost-based, fee-for-service contracts that were commonplace in the private sector.

In 1982, in virtual tandem with the private sector, Medicare became a cost-conscious payor to hospitals when it instituted the diagnosis-related group (DRG) system of payment. Diagnosis-related groups may vary from ear, nose, mouth, and throat malignancies to thyroid procedures to coronary bypass open-heart surgery. Under this reimbursement system, the government sets the price that will be paid for acute hospital care. Rehabilitation, psychiatric, children's, and sole hospital providers in rural areas are exempt from DRG reimbursement. Hospitals are paid a fixed amount to cover operating costs and a single rate for capital costs for each of 490-plus DRGs for each admitted patient. Differential payments are allowed for high-wage areas, the presence of a graduate medical education program, and for a disproportionate share of low-income patients. Outlier payments are also made for patients with "unusually" long stays or "extraordinarily" high costs [Prospective Payment Assessment Commission, *Medicare and the American Health Care System*, Report to the Congress, June 1995, Washington, DC, pp. 35, 46, 47]. Hospitals under the DRG system have incentives to reduce costs for each admission to the hospital.

The DRG system is both regulatory and competitive. The federal government fixes the rate at which Medicare patients are reimbursed. Within this rate, however, hospitals can contain costs in whichever way they choose. Rate setting in Medicare is hampered by the numerous loopholes that can arise in regulatory schemes. First, only in-patient hospital costs are regulated. Patients, therefore, may be shifted to unregulated out-patient departments. Patients may also be shifted to nursing homes or to physician offices. When individuals enter hospitals with more than one ailment falling into more than one DRG category, incentives exist for the hospital to select the DRG category which would pay the greatest reimbursement.

Although DRGs appeared to contain in-patient hospital costs, they created inefficiencies in the health care sector. At the root of many of these flaws is the presumption of the government that it can determine the price of hospital care for each of more than 490 DRGs. This would be a difficult task if the good or service purchased were as simple as, say, an umbrella. But even umbrellas come in different shades and quality, all of which can be altered in response to a government-determined price. In addition, DRG reimbursement covers in-patient costs only. Robinson has shown, for example, that the DRG payment for hospital care and a fixed-rate payment for nursing home care has created an inefficient market for nursing home care as the demand for such care has increased [James C. Robinson, "Administered Pricing and Vertical Integration in the Hospital Industry," *Journal of Law and Economics*, 39 (1996): 357–378].

Medicare hospital expenditures increased from $7.5 billion in 1970 to $36.8 billion in 1980, a 491 percent increase [U.S. Department of Commerce, *Statistical Abstract of the United States, 1994*, p. 113]. Between 1985, two years after implementation of the DRG system, and 1995, Medicare hospital expenditures increased from $72.3 billion to $181.5 billion, a 251 percent increase. Medicare out-patient expenditures, however, increased during the latter period from $4.3 billion to $15.4 billion, a 357 percent increase [U.S. Department of Commerce, *Statistical Abstract of the United States, 1997*, p. 115]. The DRG system seems to have held down in-patient Medicare expenditures as expected, but it seems to have caused some substitution of out-patient for in-patient expenditures. The increase in out-patient hospital expenditures occurred in spite of the large copayments Medicare beneficiaries have to pay. (Unlike physician services, for example, beneficiaries are responsible for 20 percent of the "hospital charge," not just 20 percent of the "Medicare-approved amount." Hence, Medicare beneficiaries, on average, are liable for 37 percent of total payments for out-patient hospital services ["Quirk in Medicare Law Yields Bigger Bills for Outpatient Care," *New York Times*, July 1, 1996, p. 1].) Home health care, also not covered by DRG reimbursement, has also shown substantial increases since 1982.

Since the DRG system applies only to Medicare patients, hospitals may shift costs to private insuring organizations, which, because of lack of bargaining power, pay full hospital charges. With the increased importance of managed care in the private sector, cost shifting has become more difficult.

It is also possible that quality of care is reduced under DRG limitations, although this may be difficult to document and quantify. Two studies have shown that there has been a 43 percent increase in those who were discharged in unstable condition in the post-DRG period from July 1985 to June 1986 compared to the pre-DRG period of calendar years 1981 and 1982 [Jacqueline Kosecoff et al., "Prospective Payment System and Impairment at Discharge," *Journal of the American Medical Association*, 264 (1990): 1980–1983; Katherine L. Kahn, "The Effects of the DRG-Based Prospective Payment System on Quality of Care for Hospitalized Medicare Patients," *Journal of the American Medical Association*, 264 (1990): 1953–1955].

In 1990, as Chapter 2 noted, Medicare began to pay physicians differently. The resource-based relative value system (RBRVS) by itself could not contain costs, but the Medicare volume performance standards (MVPS) were designed to control physician expenditures by tying physician fee updates to prior volume. Physician costs under Medicare continued to increase, however, as the MVPS was updated each year. Some have questioned the feasibility of an update based on all fees nationwide or the lumping together of all physician specialties, but since each provider alone has no incentive to contain costs, it may make little difference [John Holahan and Stephen Zuckerman, "The Future of Medicare Volume Performance Standards," *Inquiry*, 30 (1993): 235–248]. Table 6-2 shows Medicare payments for physician services for selected years, between 1980 and 1996.

Because there are different demand and supply pressures in each area for each physician specialty, some physicians are allowed to "balance bill" the

TABLE 6-2. Medicare payments for physician services in selected years, 1980–1996

Year	Physician payment (in billions of dollars)
1980	8.4
1985	17.1
1990	29.5
1991	31.4
1992	32.4
1993	34.2
1994	37.2
1995	39.7
1996	41.7

Source: Prospective Payment Assessment Commission, *Medicare and the American Health Care System*, Report to the Congress, June 1997, Table C-5, p. 137.

patient beyond the fee set by Medicare. These nonparticipating physicians may now bill up to 15 percent of the Medicare payment on a claim-by-claim basis. However, physicians who experience an exceptionally high demand for their services or believe they deliver a higher quality of care cannot realize increased financial rewards beyond the 15 percent [David C. Colby, "Balance Billing Under Medicare: Protecting Beneficiaries and Preserving Physician Participation," *Journal of Health Politics, Policy and Law*, 20 (1995): 65–74].

The Competitive Approach

The enrollment of Medicare beneficiaries in health maintenance organizations is another approach to cost containment. Beneficiaries have a choice between health maintenance organizations and fee-for-service physicians and hospitals in the hope that through competition the HMO presence will lower the costs of fee-for-service providers. However, comparatively few Medicare beneficiaries have enrolled in health maintenance organizations. As late as 1990, only 3.5 percent of the Medicare population were enrolled in HMOs [*Health Care Financing Review*, Medicare and Medicaid Statistical Supplement, February 1995, p. 24]. By 1996, however, 9.1 percent of beneficiaries were enrolled in 202 health maintenance organizations or risk-based plans [Prospective Payment Assessment Commission, *Medicare and the American Health Care System*, Report to the Congress, June 1996, Table 2-3, p. 40]. The growth in number of individuals enrolled in HMOs may be due to an increasing appeal of the scope of benefits HMOs offer as well as the absence of claim forms to be filed. It may also be due to the increasing number of HMOs in the Medicare marketplace, which offer considerable out-of-pocket savings.

Medicare HMOs may be staff or group model entities. They must each have a basic benefit package equal to at least the benefit package offered to traditional Medicare beneficiaries. Most HMOs, however, offer services beyond traditional coverage, such as no deductibles and coverage of pharmaceuticals, immunizations, and routine physicals, in order to attract members [Shoshanna Sofaer and Margo Lee-Hurwicz, "When Medical Group and HMO Part Company: Disenrollment Decisions in Medicare HMOs," *Medical Care*, 31 (1993): 808–821, p. 808; Carlos Zarabozo et al., "Medicare Managed Care: Numbers and Trends," *Health Care Financing Review*, 17 (1996): 243–261, p. 254]. Differences in premiums can reflect these differences in coverage, and, in some markets, a number of HMOs may compete against one another [Sofaer, pp. 808–809]. Zarabozo et al. report that in 1994, 56 percent of beneficiaries were able to choose between two or more Medicare managed care plans in their area, although 25 percent of Medicare HMOs are in the areas of southern California, Phoenix, and Miami [pp. 243–250].

The federal government must, even under a competitive system, still decide how much to reimburse health maintenance organizations relative to fee-for-service providers. Medicare generally reimburses each health maintenance organization at the same prospective capitation amount regardless of the quality of the plan. In order to adjust for differences in the case mix of enrollees in Medicare HMOs and enrollees who remain in fee-for-service plans, the government (Health Care Financing Administration) pays HMOs at 95 percent of the adjusted average per capita cost (AAPCC) of Medicare enrollees in traditional fee-for-service plans. Four main elements are taken into consideration in the calculation of the AAPCC. These are the age and gender mix of the population, institutional status such as hospitalization, nursing or convalescent homes (or welfare status, for someone not in an institution), and regional cost differences [Kenneth G. Manton and Eric Stallard, "Analysis of Underwriting Factors for AAPCC," *Health Care Financing Review*, 14 (1992): 117–132]. The AAPCC formula has been criticized, however, because it may only capture a small proportion of variation in health care costs [James C. Beebe, "An Outlier Pool for Medicare HMO Payments," *Health Care Financing Review*, 14 (1992): 59–63]. In addition, the formula may be too generous to health maintenance organizations if HMOs attract the lowest-risk individuals. In contrast, Frank W. Porell and Christopher P. Tompkins found that a more than a one-third decline in the number of HMOs entering into contracts with Medicare between the years 1987 and 1991 was due to possible unfavorable risk selection ["Medicare Risk Contracting: Identifying Factors Associated with Market Exit, *Inquiry*, 30 (1993): 157–169]. In part, this was due to the enrollment of a higher proportion of Medicare disabled individuals.

The calculation of a risk-adjusted measure is essential to help avoid cream skimming when two or more health care plans are in competition. If the case-mix measure is too liberal, some plans will realize supracompetitive profits. If the case-mix measure is too restrictive, HMOs will leave the marketplace. A poorly calculated AAPCC formula will mean less effective competition among HMOs and between HMOs and the fee-for-service sector. The calculation of a risk-adjusted measure is also necessary in the private sector when two or more health plans compete.

Medicare and Home Health Care

Home health care costs, the fastest-growing portion of Medicare, increased from under $3 billion in 1986 to $18.3 billion in 1996 [Prospective Payment Assessment Commission, *Medicare and the American Health Care System*, Report to the Congress, June 1997, p. 110]. Most of this increase in expenditures stems from an increase in number of visits as well as increases in number of eligible enrollees [p. 110]. In 1996 approximately 3.7 million individuals used Medicare home health care services [p. 111]. In addition, home health care services are subject to moral hazard exaggerated by few or no patient copayments [p. 110]. To be eligible for home health care benefits, beneficiaries must be, of course, homebound, need physical therapy, speech pathology, skilled nursing care, or occupational therapy, and must be under the care of a physician [Bruce C. Vladeck and Nancy A. Miller, "The Medicare Home Health Initiative," *Health Care Financing Review*, 16 (1994): 7–16]. A Medicare-approved home health agency must provide the services [p. 8].

Since home health care agencies offer an array of services, it is of interest to ascertain if there are economies of scope in the production of such services. Economies of scope are found when the costs of production of all of the services of a firm are less than the combined costs of producing each unit separately. In her study of Medicare-certified home health agencies in Connecticut during 1988–1992, Theresa I. Gonzales found that when firms performed fewer services costs decreased, but after nine services were provided, costs began to increase ["An Empirical Study of Economies of Scope in Home Healthcare," *Health Services Research*, 32 (1997): 313–323]. Thus, Gonzales concluded that many of the home health agencies in her analysis experienced diseconomies of scope. If Medicare aims to be cost conscious, and if the results of the Gonzales study can be generalized, Medicare may consider reimbursing only the home health care agencies performing fewer services. An increase in copayments may also be in order for an industry so subject to moral hazard.

State of Medicare: Summary

It has been predicted that by the year 2001, the Medicare Trust Fund, Part A, will be bankrupt. The Medicare Trust Fund, Part B, has never been designed to pay for itself, and the three-quarters of the Fund not covered by premiums adds to the federal debt. When one examines the current and future trends of the proportions of the working-age population and the Medicare beneficiary population, one observes a lower and lower ratio of the working population to the Medicare beneficiary population, which, of course, will exacerbate the problem even further. According to the calculations of the 1996 Board of Trustees of the Hospital Insurance Trust Fund, in 1995 there were 3.9 workers to pay for each Medicare beneficiary, while only 2.2 workers are projected for each Medicare beneficiary in the year 2030 and only 2.0 workers for each beneficiary in the year 2060 [The Board of Trustees, Federal Hospital Insurance Trust Fund, *1996 Annual Report of the Board of Trustees of the Federal Hospital Insurance Trust Fund*, p. 13].

One might also question the overall cost effectiveness of spending increasing amounts on Medicare when so many individuals under age 65 have no health insurance at all. Moreover, approximately 28 percent of all Medicare expenditures are for individuals who are in their last year of life [J. D. Lubitz and G. F. Riley, "Trends in Medicare Payments in the Last Year of Life," *New England Journal of Medicine*, 328, (1993): 1092–1096].

The DRG reimbursement system appears to control in-patient hospital expenditures at the expense of inefficiencies in that segment as well as inefficiencies in other segments of the health care sector. No economic theory states that the DRG system, with the government as payor of services, is superior to that of competitive bidding by the provider of services. Indeed, because Medicare does not pay each hospital differently, and has little information on each hospital's cost of services, Medicare-determined DRGs are inherently inefficient.

Medicaid

Medicaid, or Title XIX of the Social Security Act, a joint state-federal health care program, was enacted by the Congress in 1965 along with the Medicare program. The federal government pays between 50 percent and 83 percent of a state Medicaid program costs, depending on the state's per capita income [*Health Care Financing Review, Medicare and Medicaid Statistical Supplement*, February 1995, p. 117]. Medicaid does not specifically target those who are poor. Indeed, 28.7 percent of those who are below the Federal Poverty Level were not covered by Medicaid in 1992 [p. 317]. Medicaid generally covers those who are on the Aid to Families with Dependent Children (AFDC) program, aged, blind, and disabled individuals under the Federal Supplemental Security Income (SSI), and, as of 1990, all children born after September 30, 1983, in families at or below the federal poverty level [p. 112].

Medicaid covers inpatient and outpatient hospital services, physician services, laboratory and x-ray services, nursing facility services (for individuals over 21 years), early and periodic screening, diagnosis, and treatment, among other miscellaneous health care services [Paul Gurny et al., "Chapter 11: A Description of Medicaid-Covered Services," *Health Care Financing Review*, 1992 Annual Supplement, pp. 285–299]. Medicaid beneficiaries generally do not have copayments or deductibles, but Medicaid payments to providers must be such that services that are available to the general population are also available to the Medicaid population [p. 285]. Janet B. Mitchell finds in her analysis of 1977–1978 and 1984–1985 national survey data, however, that physicians are willing to treat "significantly more" patients on Medicaid the higher the Medicaid fees ["Physician Participation in Medicaid Revisited," *Medical Care*, 29 (1991): 645–653].

Medicaid has reimbursed health services in a number of ways as different states have attempted different reimbursement methods. Initially, physicians and hospitals were reimbursed on a fee-for-service basis, but since 1983, a number of growing Medicaid beneficiaries have participated in managed care or coordinated care programs. In 1983, 750,000 individuals were enrolled in Medicaid managed care plans compared to 3.6 million enrolled in 235 plans in 1992 [Gurny et al., pp. 294, 296]. By 1995, 11.6 million Medicaid beneficiaries, or 32.1 percent of the entire Medicaid population, were enrolled in managed care [Prospective Payment Assessment Commission, *Medicare and the American Health Care System*, Report to the Congress, June 1996, p. 44]. Under managed or coordinated care, Medicaid services are provided for a fixed payment per capita [Gurny et al., p. 294].

In a 1996 analysis of Medicaid capitated health maintenance organizations in the state of Florida, Joan L. Buchanan et al. found reductions in the likelihood of the use of health care services, even with some unfavorable risk selection, but no reductions in hospital utilization alone. ["Medicaid Health Maintenance Organizations: Can They Reduce Program Spending?" *Medical Care*, 34 (1996): 249–263]. This result, which is contrary to the findings of previous studies which showed reduced hospital utilization in managed care plans, may or may not be due to the large number of Medicaid enrollees who are women of child-bearing age with little discretion in hospital use.

In addition to different modes of reimbursement in each state, Medicaid has attempted a number of statewide demonstration projects in which the coverage and reimbursement mechanisms are different from those of mainstream Medicaid fee-for-service programs. For example, in Arizona, under the Arizona Health Care Cost Containment System (AHCCCS), Medicaid beneficiaries since 1982 enroll in plans that submit winning bids to the State under a competitive bidding process. Plans must be fully capitated but may pay its providers on a fee-for-service, capitation, or salary basis [Nelda McCall et al., "Managed Medicaid Cost Savings: The Arizona Experience," *Health Affairs*, 11 (1994): pp. 234–245, p. 234]. Plans must agree to provide all eligible services (including acute and long-term care). Evidence exists that for medical costs only, the AHCCCS realized a 69 percent increase in monthly per capita costs between 1983 and 1991 compared to a 113 percent increase in a number of states with traditional Medicaid programs [McCall et al., p. 243]. The reliability of comparisons of states with different populations and geographic characteristics might be questioned, however. When compared with privately insured patients, however, the hospital utilization and mortality levels of AHCCCS patients, in general (there were some exceptions in vaginal births in which length of stay was shorter and Caesarean births in which length of stay was longer), was found to be no different in a study using 1989–1990 data [Lawton R. Burns et al., "Hospital Utilization and Mortality Levels for Patients in the Arizona Health Care Cost Containment System," *Inquiry* 30 (1993): 142–156].

In California since 1982 under the Medi-Cal program, hospitals also bid for state contracts in a competitive system. Bids are on a per diem basis rather than on total hospital costs per capita. The utilization review system in the state continued to be responsible for controlling excessive utilization [Stephen T. Mennemeyer and Lois Olinger, "Selective Contracting in California: Its Effect on Hospital Finances," *Inquiry* 26 (1989): 442–457]. No adjustment was made for the case mix of any of the competing hospitals, but those with a disproportionate share of uninsured patients have more recently received a higher reimbursement rate [pp. 444–455]. In the early years of the program, Mennemeyer and his colleagues found a 19 percent reduction in per diem costs due to selective contracting [p. 455]. However, J. F. Holahan and J. W. Cohen have suggested that these early results may reflect the implementation of preadmission and concurrent review programs rather than selective contracting [*Medicaid: The Trade-Off Between Cost Containment and Access to Care* (Washington, DC: Urban Institute, 1986)].

With selective contracting one might observe a decline, over time, in per diem rates of hospitals as hospitals become more efficient. One might also see an increase in length of stay, in which hospitals may gain additional funds without losing the bid. Finally, one might observe an increase in outpatient costs that may not be covered by the per diem bid process. Based on the degree of success of utilization review programs, the number of admissions may or may not decline. Some or all of the hospitals may still make a supracompetitive profit or may deliver lower quality of care.

How might hospitals reduce costs over time? If hospitals are able to treat a greater number of patients, they may realize economies of scale in certain procedures, which can lead to lower costs. If hospitals have excess capacity (as they do in California), they also might be willing to reduce their bids, since the expense of the fixed capacity of the hospital might be reduced to the extent that hospitals can admit patients whose charges exceed the average costs of their hospital stay.

In most analyses of selective contracting, the effects of Medicaid selective contracting are intertwined with selective contracting in the private sector in the formation of preferred provider organizations (PPOs). An exception is a study by James C. Robinson and Ciaran Phibbs, who examined the results of only Medicaid selective contracting in California between 1982 and 1986 ["An Evaluation of Medicaid Selective Contracting in California," *Journal of Health Economics*, 8 (1989): 437–455]. Robinson and Phibbs found that selective contracting reduced the rate of increase in average costs of admission.

In later analyses of the selective contracting program in California, Jack Zwanziger et al. found that from 1982 to 1988, hospitals in more competitive areas experienced lower rates of increase in real expenses than hospitals in less competitive areas ["How Hospitals Practice Cost Containment with Selective Contracting and the Medicare Prospective Payment System," *Medical Care*, 32 (1994): 1153–1162]. Definitions of competition, however, can be marred by examining only the Herfindahl Index, or the sum of the market shares of the firms in the relevant geographic market used by Zwanziger et al. and other industrial organization economists. (The Herfindahl Index gives greater emphasis to the larger firms in the market. It alone cannot assess the other competitive conditions in the market, such as barriers to entry. The relevant market, however, is not easily defined and, as Chapter 3 shows, depends, in part, on an analysis of how far patients traveled for hospital care. This calculation was not made in the Zwanziger et al. analysis). More important, changes in hospital costs have little to do with the state of competition in equilibrium. Competition can enable firms to operate more efficiently, which can mean a one-time drop in hospital costs. What one observes in the Zwanziger et al. analysis is, perhaps, a continuing movement toward competition as hospitals react to the incentives of buyers that are purchasing hospital care on a per diem basis. In a later analysis of California hospitals, Zwanziger et al. found that for all purchasers, including Medicaid, hospitals in areas with greater amounts of competition had realized revenues 18 percent below those in less competitive areas between 1982 and 1990 ["Costs and Price Competition in California Hospitals, 1980–1990," *Health Affairs*, Fall 1994, pp. 118–126]. They also point out how important excess capacity is in the competitive areas, for otherwise hospitals would have little incentive to lower prices.

In another statewide program, TennCare, implemented in 1994 in the state of Tennessee, Medicaid eligibility is extended to those with preexisting conditions and those not eligible for employer-sponsored or government-sponsored plans [David R. Mirvis, "TennCare—Health System Reform for Tennesseans," *Journal of the American Medical Association*, 274 (1995): 1235–1241]. Eligible individuals choose a managed care plan in their region. There are twelve private, nonprofit, managed care organizations licensed to operate in Tennessee, but only a few may compete in some regions of the state [p. 1236]. There is an open-enrollment period once a year [p. 1236]. Managed care organizations each have a standardized benefit package that includes inpatient and outpatient services, physician services, laboratory tests, and x-rays [p. 1237]. The state of Tennessee pays each of the managed care organizations a capitated amount, and within that amount the managed care organization is expected to negotiate its own payment rates with providers. Although the percentage of individuals under age 65 with health insurance increased from 89 percent in 1993 to 95 percent in 1994 [p. 1239], the size of the capitation rate seemed to cause a low physician participation rate. As of December 1993, fewer than one-third of the state's physicians agreed to participate [p. 1240], which might have contributed to operating losses of the hospitals [p. 1239].

Medicaid Expenditures

From 1966 to 1995, total Medicaid expenditures increased from $1.3 billion to $133.1 billion—more than a 100-fold increase [Katharine R. Levit et al., "National Health Care Expenditures," *Health Care Financing Review*, 18 (1996): Tables 11–13, pp. 205–207].

Since 1989, the overall growth in Medicaid expenditures has been enormous and significantly greater than the growth in the Medicare program. There are a number of reasons for these increases. Marcia Wade and Stacy Berg ["Causes of Medicaid Expenditure Growth," *Health Care Financing Review*, 16 (1995): 11–25] suggest that the prevalence of AIDS, of which Medicaid is the most important payment source, has significantly affected Medicaid expenditures [p. 11]. Also contributing to Medicaid growth was the Boren Amendment, which required "reasonable" payments for nursing facilities and hospitals. In addition, the Omnibus Budget Reconciliation Act (OBRA; 1989) eliminated reimbursement for intermediate-care-facilities (ICFs) nursing homes; only skilled nursing facilities (SNFs) were acceptable for reimbursement. Long-term care for the disabled and the elderly accounted for 59 percent of Medicaid spending in 1994, and the increase in the number of elderly has added to the growth in Medicaid costs [Prospective Payment Assessment Commission, *Medicare and the American Health Care System*, Report to the Congress, June 1996, p. 44; also see Chapter 7]. Finally, in 1990, Medicaid coverage was expanded to provide for a greater number of disabled children (Wade and Berg, p. 12).

Regulation of Hospitals

State Hospital Rate-Setting Programs

A number of states regulated hospital rates between 1970 and 1990. Some used an all-payor system in which each payor, public and private, in the program paid the same rates; other states used a partial-payor system in which only the public payors (usually Medicare and Medicaid) paid the same rate. Stephen Zuckerman has shown that the all-payor states of New

Jersey, Maryland, New York, and Massachusetts had some short-term reductions in the growth of hospital costs compared with the partial-payor states of Connecticut, Rhode Island, Washington, and Wisconsin. ["Rate Setting and Hospital Cost-Containment: All-Payer versus Partial-Payer Approaches," *Health Services Research*, 22 (1987): 307–326]. Both the all-payor and the partial-payor states, according to Zuckerman, had lower growth in hospital costs than the unregulated states. Zuckerman did not measure changes in nonhospital costs or quality of care.

At the end of 1995, only the state of Maryland regulated hospital rates. In Maryland, rates of services delivered in an inpatient hospital setting have been regulated by the Health Services Cost Review Commission (HSCRC) since 1974. For example, in Maryland all payors, including HMOs, pay the same charges to hospitals. Early evidence (using 1977–1981 data) shows that the HSCRC, when using stringent cost-containment measures, has reduced hospital costs, but it is unknown how costs outside the hospital have been controlled [David S. Salkever et al., "Hospital Cost Efficiency under Per Service and Per Case Payment in Maryland: A Tale of the Carrot and the Stick," *Inquiry*, 23 (Spring 1986): 56–66].

Additional Regulation

In addition to the regulation of reimbursement, other attempts at regulation of hospital care have been made. States have used certificate-of-need legislation to limit the number of hospital beds, new construction of hospitals, and expansion of hospital technology [Robert B. Hackey, "New Wine in Old Bottles: Certificate of Need Enters the 1990's," *Journal of Health Politics, Policy and Law*, 18, (1993): 927–935]. The theory behind certificate-of-need legislation is that an increased supply of beds or equipment generates unnecessary utilization. However, with the advent of managed care, states have less incentive to enact certificate-of-need laws, and indeed many states have discarded such laws. Hospitals have little incentive to increase the number of beds or acquire new technology if these actions result in costs greater than those managed care plans are willing to pay hospitals.

Health Care Marketplace

Even in the public sector, one observes a movement toward market forces. Since 1982, Medicare and Medicaid have been, albeit imperfect, cost-conscious buyers of inpatient hospital services. Cost containment in health care must be weighed, as it is in all other industries, with accessibility, quality of care, and other attributes. In *Massachusetts* v. *Dukakis*, physicians contested a ban on balance billing by the state's Medicaid program. The state had an interest in holding down Medicaid costs for its citizens. In contrast, by banning balance billing, the state may have discouraged participation by higher quality physicians who received equal or higher rates of reimbursement in the private sector.

The court ruling affirmed the ban on balance billing by the state of Massachusetts. In the court's view, the state, as cost-conscious payor, could pay physicians within the guidelines of the Medicaid program. This may have meant a decline in quality of care or accessibility, but the state had the right to negotiate for the lowest price (inclusive of balance billing) and save Medicaid beneficiaries the higher charges of balance billing. Economic theory suggests that price discrimination, or the ability of the physician to charge whatever the market will bear, to various individuals in the same service would be more efficient. Budget or distribution questions, however, are factors in government policy. [For an excellent discussion of the economic theory of balance billing, see Jacob Glazer and Thomas G. McGuire, "Should Physicians Be Permitted to 'Balance Bill' Patients?" *Journal of Health Economics*, 11 (1993): 239–258.]

Chapter 6 Appendix

**Massachusetts Medical Society, et al.,
Plaintiffs, Appellants,**

v.

Michael S. Dukakis, et al., Defendants, Appellees

No. 86-1575
United States Court of Appeals,
First Circuit
Decided March 30, 1987

This case concerns the legal status of "balance billing" within the federal Medicare program. Balance billing is the practice by which a doctor bills a patient for the balance of the doctor's fee over and above the amount that the Medicare program has determined to be a "reasonable charge." Massachusetts has enacted a statute that forbids balance billing (p. 790).

The Act provides two mechanisms by which the Secretary of Health and Human Services—or to be more accurate, a Medicare insurance carrier—may pay a doctor for treatment of a Medicare beneficiary:

[P]ayment will ... be made [by the carrier] (i) on the basis of an itemized bill; or (ii) on the basis of an assignment under the terms of which ... the reasonable charge is the full charge for the service (p. 792).

Under either payment method, HHS pays 80 percent of the reasonable charge for the doctor's services. If the doctor chooses the second payment method and accepts "assignment" of the patient's right to payment, the Medicare carrier will pay him directly 80 percent of the reasonable charge. In addition, the doctor may bill his patient for the remaining 20 percent of the reasonable charge. But, he may not balance bill—he may not bill his patient for more than the reasonable charge.

If the doctor instead chooses the first method of payment—if he submits an "itemized bill" to his patient—the patient will submit the doctor's bill and a claim for payment to the Medicare carrier, and the carrier will pay the patient 80 percent of the reasonable charge (pp. 792–793).

Under this method, the patient under ordinary contract law would have to pay the doctor's fee including any excess over that reasonable charge. In effect, a doctor who chooses assignment billing accepts the reasonable charge ceiling as a quid pro quo for assured direct payment from the government of 80 percent of that reasonable charge (p. 793).... And, in effect, a doctor who chooses itemized billing accepts the risk of nonpayment or late payment by the patient in exchange for the "option" (as MMS [Massachusetts Medical Society, the American Medical Association, and an

89

individual Massachusetts doctor collectively] puts it) to charge more than the reasonable charge. MMS says that the words "itemized bill," taken in context, create a statutory right to balance bill (p. 793).

We are similarly unconvinced by MMS's efforts to prove factually in the district court that the Massachusetts balance billing ban will create an "obstacle" to providing needy patients with access to care. By putting various factual assumptions to experts, counsel elicited testimony that the ban could cause as many as ten to twenty percent of the Massachusetts doctors who formerly treated Medicare patients to stop doing so. Yet, it is undisputed that 99 percent of all Massachusetts doctors participate in Blue Shield, which has had such a ban since the mid-1960s (p. 795).

MMS argues that the condition that Massachusetts imposes on medical licensees—a promise not to balance bill—is not rationally connected with a doctor's "fitness or capacity to practice" medicine (p. 797).

In our view, however, this "promise" simply amounts to a rule. It is a rule that forbids balance billing. And, there is nothing irrational about a state's saying that a doctor, entering the profession, must promise to follow the rules (p. 797). Nor is it irrational to say that a doctor who seriously violates the rule—who commits a violation that is "commensurate with" the penalty of license revocation—is not "fit" to practice medicine (p. 797).

For these reasons, the judgment of the district court is Affirmed (p. 797).

7
Long-Term Care Industry

The long-term care industry consists of health care services, social services, and residential services provided to disabled or elderly persons over a long period of time. Disabilities may be due to physical disease, severe mental disease, trauma, or mental retardation.

Long-term care expenditures are the fastest-growing portion of the health care sector. Between 1985 and 1995, for example, nursing home expenditures more than doubled, from $30.7 billion to $77.9 billion [Katharine R. Levit et al., "National Health Expenditures, 1995," *Health Care Financing Review*, 18 (1996): 175–214, Table 9, p. 201]. Approximately 95 percent of long-term care expenditures were reimbursements for institutional care (nursing homes, intermediate care facilities for the mentally retarded, and mental hospitals), with the remainder going for home health care [J. F. Holahan and J. W. Cohen, *Medicaid: The Trade-Off Between Cost Containment and Access to Care* (Washington, DC: Urban Institute, 1987)]. Moreover, as Christine E. Bishop points out ["Competition in the Market for Nursing Home Care," in *Competition in the Health Care Sector: Ten Years Later*, ed. W. Greenberg (Durham, NC: Duke University Press, 1988), pp. 119–38], more than 70 percent of individuals who need long-term care assistance live in their own homes and receive most of their aid from family and friends. William J. Scanlon ["Possible Reforms for Financing Long-Term Care," *Journal of Economic Perspectives*, 6 (Summer 1992): 43–58] shows that 80 percent of the disabled elderly and 41 percent of severely disabled individuals live at home.

The long-term care industry should grow even faster in the future because those over the age of 65 are the fastest-growing segment of the U.S. population. In addition, the fastest-growing portion of the 65-and-older group is the oldest segment—people over the age of 85. In 1995, there were approximately 33.6 million individuals over the age of 65 and 3.6 million individuals over the age of 85, or 12.6 percent and 1.3 percent of the total population, respectively. By the year 2030, there will be approximately 70 million individuals over the age of 65 and approximately 9 million individuals over the age of 85, or 20.1 percent and 2.5 percent of the population, respectively [U.S. Department of Commerce, *Statistical Abstract of the United States, 1995*, Table 17, p. 17].

Individuals who are older than 85 are much more likely to need assisted care than those between the ages of 65 and 85. Fewer than 40 percent of nursing home residents aged 65 to 74 had difficulty in eating, while approximately 56 percent of residents aged 85 and older needed assistance in eating [M. G. Kovar, G. Hendershot, and E. Mathis, "Older People in the United States Who Receive Help with Basic Activities of Daily Living," *American Journal of Public Health*, 79 (1989): 778–779]. According to Kovar, Hendershot, and Mathis, about 88 percent of nursing home residents are elderly. The remainder are blind, disabled, or retarded.

Using survey data from a national sample of adults above age 25 who died in 1986, Peter Kemper and Christopher M. Murtaugh found that the probability of individuals eventually entering a nursing home is significant, as are substantial lengths of stay ["Lifetime Use of Nursing Home Care," *New England Journal of Medicine*, 324 (1991): 595–600]. In 1986, 29 percent of those who died after age 25 had been residents of a nursing home and nearly one-half of these individuals had spent at least one year in a nursing home during their lifetime. For those who had turned 65 in 1990, Kemper and Murtaugh predicted that 43 percent would enter a nursing home and 55 percent of those would spend more than a year there.

An increase in the number of people who are very old and disabled will shift the demand curve for long-term care to the right. This upward pressure of demand should increase prices and utilization of long-term care institutions and stimulate investments in new facilities, provided there are no governmental restrictions in pricing or barriers to entry of new and existing firms.

Economic Attributes of the Long-Term Care Industry

Several economic attributes make an analysis of the behavior of the long-term care industry different from that of the acute care industry. The first is the limited role of the physician in long-term care. In long-term care, the physician has a passive role; he or she does not ordinarily have the main responsibility for referring individuals to or placing them in nursing homes or home health care agencies. The physician does not control the length of stay in nursing homes. Physicians rarely use new technology—which is responsible for so large a proportion of acute care costs—for long-term care purposes.

Second, long-term care is custodial rather than curative. It may include assistance with bathing, eating, and dressing. Nursing home stays average more than 600 days, compared to fewer than 7 days in a hospital [Kovar, Hendershot, and Mathis, 1989]. Once an illness in hospitals is contained, individuals are discharged. Individuals in long-term care facilities are less likely to return to an environment in which assistance is not required.

Third, the types and scope of third-party coverage are different for acute and long-term care. In acute care, in 1995, Medicare accounted for 32.2 percent of hospital expenditures and 19.8 percent of physician expenditures, while Medicaid accounted for 14.8 percent and 7.1 percent of hospital and physician expenditures, respectively. Private health insurance, in contrast, accounted for approximately 32.3 percent of expenditures for hospital services and 48.1 percent of expenditures for physician services. Patients and other private sources accounted for 6.5 percent and 20.2 percent of hospital and physician expenditures, respectively [Levit et al., Tables 12 and 13, pp. 206–207]. For nursing home care expenditures, however, Medicaid in 1995 paid 46.5 percent, while Medicare paid 9.4 percent, private insurance paid 3.3 percent, and individuals paid 36.7 percent. The remainder came from miscellaneous private and public sources [Levit et al., Table 14, p. 208]. For long-term care as a whole, data from the Employee Benefit Research Institute (EBRI) ["Long-Term Care and the Private Insurance Market," *EBRI Issue Brief 163*, July 1995, Chart 1, p. 6] show that in 1993 Medicaid paid 43.4 percent of expenditures while Medicare paid approximately 15.7 percent, private insurance paid 4.7 percent, and individuals paid approximately 30.2 percent. Six percent came from miscellaneous private and public sources.

The limited insurance coverage of long-term care services relative to acute care services may reduce the utilization of long-term care services where benefits are less than societal cost. However, insured long-term care services, because they reduce financial responsibilities of the patient for daily living, are subject to moral hazard, perhaps to a greater degree than acute care services. Many elderly individuals could justify some assistance in bathing or dressing, for example, if these activities were covered by insurance. As we shall see, however, individuals are reluctant to purchase long-term care insurance.

The determinants of long-term care utilization derive not only from an individual's need for services but also from demographics and the mores of society. A large number of individuals who, in years past, might have stayed home to care for their parents are now in the formal labor force, which increases the opportunity cost of attending to the needs of elderly parents. In addition, divorce rates have grown, and individuals are unlikely to care for a former spouse's parents. At the same time, more families have two working members and are better able to afford professional long-term care services for their relatives.

There are also information asymmetries between the nursing home and the disabled or elderly individual. Although individuals may have assistance from family and friends in selecting a nursing home, they may have a difficult time judging the quality of care provided once they are admitted. Moreover, once a person is situated in a nursing home, substantial mental, physical, and financial costs are attached to moving the person to another home. For most other goods and services in the economy, even though there may be information asymmetries between seller and buyer, at least there is a finite end to the mistake: if one buys an inferior automobile it can be sold; if one eats in poor restaurant, one never eats there again. The selection of an unsuitable nursing home may not be so easily corrected.

Long-Term Care Insurance

Medicaid

Medicaid pays for skilled, intermediate, custodial care and some assisted living care, home care, and community-based long-term care, depending in which state the patient resides [EBRI, p. 7]. To be eligible for Medicaid, one has to meet the criteria for all Medicaid programs discussed in Chapter 6.

When assets fall below a certain level, or when income each year falls below a certain level, an individual is eligible for Medicaid. This is called "spenddown." The amount of assets or income that must be depleted before Medicaid pays for care depends on the state in which one resides, the amount of housing that can be counted in total assets, and the extent of monetary allowance for the non-Medicaid spouse. This may be viewed as a large copayment prior to the use of Medicaid catastrophic insurance. Transferring assets to a spouse prior to admittance to a nursing home has become more difficult since the Omnibus Budget Reconciliation Act of 1993 restricted such transfers [Korbin Liu et al., "Medicaid Spenddown in Nursing Homes," *The Gerontologist*, 30 (1990): 7–15; EBRI, pp. 7–8]. Indeed, Frank A. Sloan and May W. Shayne have found that most disabled elderly are available for nursing home benefits when entering a home because comparatively few have sufficient assets and income ["Long-Term Care, Medicaid, and Impoverishment of the Elderly," *Milbank Quarterly*, 17 (1993): 575–599].

Medicaid is the largest purchaser of long-term care services. As such it is a monopsony buyer. It pays rates for nursing home residents far below those of other payors; higher rates can be collected from private individuals and private health insurers. Thus, nursing homes are reluctant to accept Medicaid patients. Since Medicaid accounts for a large share of nursing home expenditures, Medicaid policies can substantially affect the viability of the nursing home industry. For example, state Medicaid plans that pay a flat, per diem fee have experienced a much lower rate of cost increases than those that pay retrospectively [John F. Holohan, "State Rate-Setting and Its Effects on the Cost of Nursing Home Care," *Journal of Health Politics, Policy and Law*, 9 (1985): 647–667]. If Medicaid fees are set too low or if they fail to consider the case mix of nursing home residents and the amount of nursing assistance the residents require, some nursing homes may not survive unless they can raise fees to private-pay patients, limit access to Medicaid, or reduce quality of care.

Medicare

Medicare covers stays in skilled nursing facilities (SNFs) that are medically necessary but only within thirty days of a hospital stay. Medicare also covers home health care if the plan of treatment is reviewed and approved by a physician. Hospice care is covered as well. In general, however, Medicare coverage does not extend to custodial, long-term care [*Health Care Financing Review*, Medicare and Medicaid Statistical Supplement, February 1995, pp. 4–5].

Private Long-Term Care Insurance

Very few individuals have private long-term care insurance. At the end of 1993, only 3.4 million policies had been sold, an increase, however, over the 815,000 policies that had been sold up to 1987 [EBRI, p. 8]. There appear to be several reasons for the relatively few long-term care policies compared to policies for acute care needs. First, individuals may place a greater value on current rather than future potentially expensive needs. They may not be interested in purchasing insurance unlikely to benefit them until as many as 20 to 50 years in the future. The uncertainty of the costs of long-term care facilities and the demand for such facilities add another cost of risk to the insurance premium. Second, the presence of Medicaid may contribute to this reluctance. Some individuals may look at Medicaid as a safety net for long-term care in case they do not have sufficient funds or insurance in their old age. Economists have suggested that, in the same way, the prospect of Social Security income in one's old age may have reduced savings by nonelderly individuals [Martin Feldstein, "Social Security, Induced Retirement, and Aggregate Capital Accumulation," *Journal of Political Economy*, 82 (1974): 905–926]. Third, those most interested in buying long-term care insurance may be excluded by preexisting conditions or may find the premiums for those near retirement age to be prohibitively expensive.

The potential of a more accessible and higher-quality nursing home may encourage individuals to purchase private long-term care insurance that allow them to make higher payments than Medicaid to nursing homes. In contrast, Susan L. Ettner finds diminished access for Medicaid patients to nursing home care ["Do Elderly Medicaid Patients Experience Reduced Access to Nursing Home Care?" *Journal of Health Economics*, 11 (1993): 259–280].

Employer-Based Long-Term Care Insurance

It is interesting to compare the number of individuals who receive long-term care insurance from their employer with the number who receive their traditional health insurance from their employer. In 1993, approximately 400,000 long-term care policies were sold through employers out of a total of 3,417,000 policies overall, or less than 12 percent of total policies sold [EBRI, pp. 8–9], in spite of the high administrative and marketing costs of private long-term care insurance. In contrast, as we have seen, more than 90 percent of individuals who have traditional health insurance receive it from their employer (see Chapter 5).

It appears that the uncertain tax status of employer-sponsored long-term care insurance is an important reason that the proportion of employer-sponsored long-term care insurance is so low. At best, the status has been ambiguous enough to prompt President Clinton to specifically include exemption of employer-paid premiums from taxes for long-term care insurance as part of his ill-fated health care reforms [Joshua M. Wiener et al., *Sharing the Burden* (Washington, DC: Brookings Institution, 1994), p. 82; Anne Marie Walsh, "Clearing Up a Murky Tax Issue," *Best's Review*, 92 (January, 1992): 41–44, 92, 93].

One lesson for long-term care insurace is that employer-sponsored health insurance would not be so pervasive if it were not for its exemption from taxes. Proposals to exempt employer-sponsored long-term care from taxes should have been resisted if the same inefficiencies found in the purchase of traditional health insurance were to be avoided [see Mark V. Pauly, "Should Long-Term Care Receive Tax Subsidies, or Is Medicaid Enough?" in *Financing Long Term Care*, ed. Mark V. Pauly and Peter Zweifel (Washington, DC: American Enterprise Institute, 1996)]. (Unfortunately, under the Kassebaum-Kennedy Bill of 1996, employer-paid long-term care insurance was made exempt from taxes.)

Nature of the Demand Facing Nursing Homes

Nursing homes face a downward sloping demand curve of individuals for services as well as the elastic demand curve of Medicaid for its services. It will always be in the interest of the nursing home, therefore, to admit higher-paying private sector patients before lower-paying Medicaid patients. Thus, "excess demand" in the form of waiting lists for long-term care exists. Occupancy rates in nursing homes are high, averaging 91.5 percent in 1991 [U.S. Department of Commerce, *Statistical Abstract of the United States*, 1995, Table 201, p. 134]. This may result in suboptimal care, patients spending unnecessary time in the hospital waiting to be admitted to nursing homes, and reduced admissions, in general, to nursing homes. Excess demand is exacerbated by a restriction in building nursing home beds (under the certificate-of-need laws) in many states [James D. Reschovsky, "Demand for and Access to Institutional Long-Term Care: The Role of Medicaid in Nursing Home Markets," *Inquiry*, 33 (1996): 15–29].

Supply of Long-Term Care Institutions

There were approximately 33,006 nursing and related care facilities in the United States in 1991 with an average of 58 beds per facility [U.S. Department of Commerce, *Statistical Abstract of the United States*, 1996, Table 205, p. 136]. Unlike most hospitals, most nursing homes are for-profit entities, with a minority owned by religious groups and other nonprofit institutions. More than 40 percent of for-profit as well as nonprofit nursing homes are members of chains (Bishop, 1988). Except for state certificate-of-need regulations that restrict the number of beds or nursing homes in an area, there do not appear to be barriers to entry to firms that would like to enter the nursing home industry.

Nursing homes compete on the basis of price, quality, and avoidance of high-risk, older individuals who might consume more services. Firms often use price discrimination in efforts to maximize profits. Since state Medicaid programs pay only at or below the competitive rate, nursing homes usually charge self-paying patients or commercial insurers a higher price. High occupancy rates (generally exceeding 90 percent) have apparently decreased nursing homes' incentive to compete on the basis of quality and dissemination of information on their quality attributes [John A. Nyman, "Excess Demand, Consumer Rationality, and the Quality of Care in Regulated Nursing Homes," *Health Services Research*, 24 (1989): 105–127]. In an excess demand market, shopping for a nursing home based on quality considerations may not be an option for many Medicaid patients. Firms, therefore, appear to compete on a quality basis only in areas where nursing home occupancy rates are relatively low. Similar to acute care hospitals, nursing homes also have incentives to admit individuals who, at least at the beginning of their stay, have less need for costly care.

There are very few studies on the profitability of nursing homes. Ronald J. Vogel, in his review of such studies performed in the 1970s ["The Industrial Organization of the Nursing Home Industry," in *Long-Term Care Perspectives from Research and Demonstrations*, ed. R. J. Vogel and H. C. Palmer (Washington, DC: U.S. Department of Health and Human Services, 1989), pp. 579–624], suggests that there appears to be "large variability" in profit rates among firms. Vogel suggests that higher profits may be due to reduced competition in some areas because of certificate-of-need regulations and that lower profits may be due to periods of rapid growth of nursing homes in some areas or to the government as a monopsonistic buyer. Nursing homes that have a greater number of self-paying patients may have a higher rate of return, especially if there are certificate-of-need or other requirements to deter new entry. There do not appear to be any economies of scale in the size of nursing homes, however, that might have enabled higher than competitive rates of return (Bishop, 1988).

Long-Term Care Alternatives to Nursing Homes

Capitated, comprehensive health care plans are a growing segment of long-term care. Like acute care, comprehensive care takes many forms, of which continuing care retirement communities (CCRCs) and social/health maintenance organizations (S/HMOs) are prominent examples. In both acute and long-term care settings, the objective of comprehensive plans is to restrict utilization to its lowest-care alternatives consistent with established standards for the quality of care. As in acute care, the lowest-cost long-term care setting may be the most comfortable as well as the least expensive one for the patient. Moreover, incentives exist in the capitated, comprehensive health plans to provide quality care both to discourage enrollees from leaving the plans and, perhaps more importantly, to encourage nonmembers to enroll.

Continuing care retirement communities are prepaid, long-term care organizations that provide residential units, social services, and nursing home facilities for their residents. Individuals usually pay a fee upon enrollment and a monthly membership fee thereafter. As of the mid-1980s, more than 100,000 individuals had enrolled in approximately 600 CCRCs [H. S. Ruchlin, "Continuing Care Retirement Communities: An Analysis of Financial Viability and Health Care Coverage," *The Gerontologist*, 28 (1988): 156–162]. Thus far, however, there have been no studies of the quality of care CCRCs deliver or the extent to which they can control long-term care costs.

Similar to the competitive effect of health maintenance organizations on the fee-for-service sector that appears to have taken place in acute care, alternatives to nursing homes may provide competition to nursing homes. Frank A. Sloan et al. examined continuing care retirement communities as an alternative to nursing home care ["Continuing Care Retirement Communities: Prospects for Reducing Institutional Long-Term Care," *Journal of Health Politics, Policy and Law*, 20 (1995): 75–98]. Sloan et al. concluded that the presence of CCRCs can contain the use of nursing home services.

Social/health maintenance organizations (integrated case-management systems) began providing services in 1983 under a Health Care Financing Administration (HCFA) demonstration project in four locations: Portland, Oregon; Brooklyn, Minneapolis, and Long Beach, California. S/HMOs differ from CCRCs in that S/HMOs provide Medicare-covered acute care services but with no copayments or deductibles. In addition, there is no apartment-living component in S/HMOs as there are in CCRCs. In both CCRCs and S/HMOs, however, a single provider is responsible for all of the care under a prospective budget and is at risk for costs exceeding this budget. S/HMOs include all of the acute care services provided under traditional HMOs as well as chronic care benefits.

A. M. Rivlin and J. M. Wiener [*Caring for the Disabled Elderly: Who Will Pay?* (Washington, DC: Brookings Institution, 1988)] have suggested that adequate enrollment has generally been a problem for S/HMOs since individuals prefer to remain with their own physician. R. Newcomer, C. Harrington, and A. Friedlob, in their examination of the HCFA project ["Social Health Maintenance Organizations: Assessing their Initial Experience," *Health Services Research*, 25 (1990): 425–454], also found disappointing enrollments, perhaps due to competition from HMOs, suboptimal marketing, and the limited size of their geographic market area. Thus far, there have been no studies on the extent to which S/HMOs may or may not be able to contain costs. However, members of S/HMOs who have completed one year in the plan appear to be no less satisfied than those in the Medicare fee-for-service program [Robert Newcomer et al., "Health Plan Satisfaction and Risk of Disenrollment Among Social/HMO and Fee-for-Service Recipients," *Inquiry*, 33 (1996): 144–154].

Another form of comprehensive care, Life Care at Home, emphasizes noninstitutional, home-based care for the elderly. Services include skilled nursing care, home-delivered meals, respite care, and pharmacy and emergency services. Acute health care benefits are an option. The Life Care at Home model may be less expensive than the CCRC model because subscribers are encouraged to live in their own homes as long as possible, a feature most elderly prefer [E. J. Tell, M. A. Cohen, and S. S. Wallack, "Life Care at Home: A New Model for Financing and Delivering Long-Term Care," *Inquiry*, 24 (1987): 245–252].

Long-Term Care in the Future

The pressures for the increased number of long-term care services that an aging population will demand suggest that there will be a continuing increase in the variety and number of different forms of long-term care. Total expenditures for long-term care will increase. The public policy challenge will be to finance the most efficient forms of long-term care without increasing the costs associated with the moral hazard of the care.

Currently, Medicaid, as the largest payor, reimburses primarily for nursing home care, which creates a reimbursement system sustaining many people in nursing homes who could be cared for at home in a less costly manner; at the same time, many disabled adults at home should be attended to in a nursing home setting but are not able to secure a room. State governments, however, may secure Medicaid waivers that may reimburse for home care and community-based care for those who should have institutionalization [J. W. Meltzer, "Financing Long-Term Care: A Major Obstacle to Reform," in *The Economics and Ethics of Long-term Care and Disability*, ed. S. Sullivan and M. E. Lewin (Washington, DC: American Enterprise Institute, 1988), pp. 56–72].

Integrated case-management plans have incentives to place individuals in the least costly setting. In addition, as Bishop (1988) points out, the integrated firms have an advantage over individuals in controlling costs in the nursing home. This is because the integrated firm has more bargaining power than a single individual as well as more information, based on a large number of patients and on the prices and qualities of various homes. Alternatively, because of moral hazard, higher long-term costs may result. If S/HMOs or other integrated plans were to compete, incentives for cream skimming would arise as they do in acute care. Indeed, a large part of the argument for government intervention in this industry is private insurers' potential avoidance of high-risk individuals.

Health Care Marketplace

In *U.S.* v. *Montana Nursing Home Association* [Federal Register, vol. 47, no. 112, Thursday, June 10, 1982, pp. 25222–25223], the Department of Justice brought suit against the Montana Nursing Home Association, a group of nursing homes that had boycotted a public entity, Medicaid. According to the June 13, 1980, Department of Justice complaint, seventy nursing homes were members of the association, which comprised more than two-thirds of all nursing home beds in Montana. It is not surprising that the nursing home association attempted to boycott Medicaid, since the fees paid by Medicaid are typically much lower than the fees paid by private payors.

Chapter 7 Appendix

United States
v.
Montana Nursing Home Association, Inc.

U.S. District Court, District of Montana,
Helena Division
No. CV-80-92-H
Entered July 1, 1982
Case No. 2771
A consent decree

• • • • •

Defendant is enjoined from:

(A) Participating in any concerted refusal by nursing homes to enter into Medicaid standard provider contracts or to participate in the Medicaid program;

(B) Participating in any agreement, understanding, plan or course of conduct with the purpose of foreseeable effect that nursing homes (1) jointly accept or reject all or any terms of Medicaid standard provider contracts; (2) jointly reject or discharge Medicaid patients; or (3) jointly threaten not to participate in the Medicaid program;

(C) Advocating or recommending that nursing home(s) (1) accept or reject all or any terms of Medicaid standard provider contracts; (2) reject or discharge Medicaid patients; or (3) threaten not to participate in the Medicaid program;

(D) Causing or permitting at any formal or informal meeting of Defendant or its committees any course of conduct or discussion of any plan having the purpose or foreseeable effect that nursing home(s) (1) jointly accept or reject all or any terms of Medicaid standard provider contracts; (2) jointly reject or discharge Medicaid patients; or (3) jointly threaten not to participate in the Medicaid program; and

(E) Nothing in this Section IV shall prohibit Defendant from:

(1) discussing or distributing factual information concerning the Medicaid program or proposed changes therein;

(2) giving fair and reasonable constructions of the terms of existing or proposed Medicaid standard provider contracts, governmental regulations, or policies and procedures relating thereto;

(3) advocating proposed changes in the Medicaid program to, or discussing the Medicaid program with, any governmental body or member or employee thereof; or

(4) seeking through any bona fide judicial or administrative law proceeding a determination of the rights or responsibilities of its members under the Medicaid program; so long as such conduct is not part of an agreement, plan or conspiracy to engage in the conduct proscribed in subsections A through D of this Section IV (pp. 72253–72254).

8
Antitrust in the Health Care Sector

The aim of the nation's antitrust laws is to promote competition within industries. Economic theory suggests that the greater the number of firms within an industry and the fewer the impediments to firms that would like to enter the industry, the more competitive the industry will be. The behavior of firms within industries may also indicate the extent of competition. For example, price collusion among firms indicates a lack of competition in an industry. Exclusion of new entrants by firms that are already in the industry may also be anticompetitive: it reduces the number of potential competitors.

Antitrust legislation is essential to a competitive environment in health care. The first antitrust law, the Sherman Act, enacted in 1890, was a response to the oil and tobacco trusts. These industries were believed to have fewer firms and higher prices than would have been the case if anticompetitive behavior, such as collusion, were prohibited.

Under Section 1 of the Sherman Act, "[E]very contract, combination in the form of trust or otherwise, or conspiracy, in restraint of trade or commerce ... is illegal." Section 2 of the act states that "every person who shall monopolize, or attempt to monopolize, or combine or conspire with any other person or persons, to monopolize any part of the trade or commerce ... shall be deemed guilty."

Two additional major antitrust laws have been passed since the Sherman Act. Major provisions of the Clayton Act, passed in 1914, were intended to prohibit price discrimination in which sellers "discriminate in price between different purchasers of commodities of like grade and quality" (Section 2) and to eliminate mergers that "lessen competition or tend to create a monopoly" (Section 7). Price discrimination was alleged to give larger buyers an unfair advantage over smaller buyers. Anticompetitive mergers might reduce the number of competitors, thereby lessening competition and creating a monopoly.

The Federal Trade Commission Act was also passed in 1914. Section 5 of this act forbade "unfair methods of competition" and created a new agency, the Federal Trade Commission, to help enforce the antitrust laws. Antitrust suits may be brought both by the Federal Trade Commission and by the U.S. Department of Justice, although only the Justice Department can bring suits that involve the Sherman Act. Private plaintiffs and state antitrust authorities may also bring antitrust suits, although these suits tend to be of less importance.

Consistent with the notion of a competitive health care system is the expectation that an increase in the supply of sellers not only brings lower prices to consumers but improves consumer welfare. An increased number of sellers—such as physicians and hospitals—brings a more efficient allocation of resources, improved quality of care, greater innovation and technology, greater access to providers, and a greater variety of services for consumers. This expected result of increased supply is not unlike the expectations in other sectors of the economy when antitrust actions are brought.

An increased supply of providers is directly antithetical to a health care regulatory environment that limits the number of beds or number of hospitals. Nonetheless, in many states that have had certificate-of-need laws, planning agencies attempted to restrict the number of new hospital beds or have reduced the number of already existing beds.

Crucial to the assumption that an increased number of competitors improves the welfare of consumers is the presence of knowledgeable buyers and demanders of goods and services. That is, a belief in the notion of consumer sovereignty is a requisite to the proposition that antitrust has a role to play in the health care sector. Demand in the health care sector arises, however, mostly from third-party payors, or managed care firms, not individual patients. Antitrust policy is therefore directed toward ensuring that third-party payors can act as cost-conscious buyers in the purchase of health care without boycotts or interference from providers. For services that are uninsured, individuals are expected to compare prices and quality of providers as they would for any other good or service.

Information on the quality and price of services offered by health care providers is fundamental to an effective antitrust policy if third parties and individuals are to act as informed buyers. To the extent that physicians can create their own demand because of uninformed patients—or managed care firms cannot assess the relative price and quality of medical and nonmedical providers, antitrust laws will be less effective.

Legal and Economic Impediments to Antitrust Policy in the Health Care Sector

Until 1975, due to legal impediments and a number of economic factors, there were few antitrust suits brought in the health care sector. Perhaps the most important legal obstacle was the belief that the health care professions were exempt from antitrust legislation because of their status as "learned professions." In *Goldfarb* v. *Virginia State Bar* [421 US 773 (1975)], however, the court found that the learned professions were not exempt from antitrust scrutiny. In this case, the Supreme Court found that the Virginia state bar association was in violation of Section 1 of the Sherman Act for setting minimum fee schedules.

A second obstacle to antitrust enforcement was the McCarran-Ferguson Act [15 USC (1945), 1011–1015], which was once interpreted to exempt insuring organizations from antitrust prosecution. Gradually, however, the courts interpreted the McCarran-Ferguson Act to apply only to the actual business of insurance firms, such as the underwriting of risks, rather than to insuring organizations and their relationships to health care providers.

Finally, many health care organizations—most hospitals, Blue Cross and Blue Shield insurance plans, and some nursing homes—are nonprofit firms. Section 4 of the Federal Trade Commission Act limits Federal Trade Commission jurisdiction to the corporation "organized to carry on business for its own profit or that of its members," although the Justice Department is not prohibited from bringing antitrust suits against nonprofit firms. Moreover, the Federal Trade Commission has suggested that nonprofit organizations can indirectly benefit for-profit providers with whom they are affiliated. For example, the Bureau of Economics of the Federal Trade Commission [*Staff Report on Physician Control of Blue Shield Plans* (Washington, DC: U.S. Government Printing Office, 1979)] argued that the nonprofit Blue Shield plan existed for the benefit of the profit-making physicians on its board. Subsequent to this report, all Blue Shield plans voluntarily eliminated physician-controlled boards.

In addition to legal barriers, economic considerations contributed to the low level of antitrust activity in health care. A relatively scarce supply of physicians, until the 1970s, made it less likely, for example, that hospitals would deny staff privileges to physicians. On the demand side, third-party payors, until the early 1980s, usually paid the bill for health care providers' services without concern about the cost of the services or number of services performed. Third-party payors, in short, were not cost-conscious buyers of health care; there was little reason for providers to resist third-party payment mechanisms.

Antitrust litigation in health care can be divided into cases that have attempted to affect demand by enabling third parties to be more cost-conscious buyers of health care and cases that have attempted to affect supply by increasing the number and variety of providers.

Antitrust and the Demand Side

As we saw in Chapter 2, economists have had an ongoing debate about whether an increase in the number of providers leads to an increase in prices or an increase in number of services rendered. One aspect of this

106   8. Antitrust in the Health Care Sector

debate is whether physicians can create their own demand or set their own price, or whether hospitals can be filled with unnecessary admissions.

This debate arises because of the possible asymmetry of information between the provider and the consumer of medical care. Providers are the experts in medical care, and patients generally lack information on the types of procedures and tests to be used. Third-party payors, however, have the ability to monitor providers because of the data they accumulate from insuring large numbers of patients. It is essential for cost containment, therefore, that third-party payors (1) secure information from providers on utilization and prices and (2) be able to contain costs without hindrance by providers.

A 1930s case brought by the U.S. Department of Justice, *U.S. v. Oregon State Medical Society* [343 US 326 (1952)], shows the early importance of utilization review by third-party insurers in their attempts to contain costs. In that case, insurers monitored the decisions of physicians to hospitalize patients, to extend the length of the hospital stay, and to determine which tests were to be performed. Physicians, however, began to resist reviews by the third-party payers. Physicians began their own health insurance plan, Oregon Physicians' Service (OPS), the forerunner to the current Blue Shield plan in Oregon, in an attempt to control utilization-review efforts by other third-party insurers. After the formation of OPS, physicians refused reimbursement by other third-party insurers because they could always rely on reimbursement by OPS. The cost-containing activities of the insurers were consequently eliminated.

The Justice Department brought suit against the Oregon State Medical Society, eight county medical societies, and eight physicians for violating Sections 1 and 2 of the Sherman Act by attempting to exclude the insurers performing cost containment from the market. Since the three largest private insurers had not been excluded and no overt action by providers to boycott insurers was found, the Supreme Court ruled 7 to 1 in 1952 that the Oregon State Medical Society had not engaged in anticompetitive behavior. The ability of the physicians to thwart utilization-review attempts by insurers discouraged utilization review by third-party firms for decades. Subsequent boycotts by provider groups were, however, found to be in violation of the antitrust laws.

The Federal Trade Commission brought suits against the Indiana Dental Association [93 FTC 392 (1979)] and the Indiana Federation of Dentists [101 FTC 57 (1983), rev'd. 745 F. 2d 1124 (7th Cir. 1984), rev'd. 476 US 447 (1986)] because the dentists in Indiana refused to furnish x-rays to third-party payors such as Aetna and Prudential who desired to contain costs. In dentistry, unlike most of medicine, there can be a time lag between diagnosis and procedure. Dental insurers, therefore, may require x-rays before authorizing treatment and then, after consulting dentists on their staffs, disapprove payment for some of the dental procedures. In Indiana, however, dentists collectively declined to comply with the x-ray requirement. The Texas Dental Association [100 FTC 536 (1982)] also hindered the cost-containment programs of third-party payors when, together with its members, it refused to furnish x-rays and other diagnostic information to third-party payors.

Both the Indiana Dental Association and the Texas Dental Association agreed in consent orders with the Federal Trade Commission not to obstruct third-party cost-containment efforts or to coerce insurers into using association-approved independent dental consultants. (A consent order, which provides for some remedial action but does not determine guilt or innocence, is not uncommon in antitrust cases.) *FTC* v. *Indiana Federation of Dentists* was eventually decided by the U.S. Supreme Court, which found that the conspiracy to withhold x-rays was in restraint of trade. The federation's arguments that insurers interfered in the dentist-patient relationship and curtailed professional prerogatives were not persuasive to the court.

In addition to cases that involve third-party attempts to review utilization, there have also been attempts by third parties to contain the fees of providers. In 1979, the Federal Trade Commission brought suit against the Michigan State Medical Society [101 FTC 191 (1983)], which had allegedly interfered with the reimbursement policies of the commercial insurers, Blue Shield of Michigan, and the state Medicaid authorities. The Commission ruled that the boycott of the insuring organizations by the medical society had the effect of decreasing competition among insuring organizations, with the result of higher fees to patients. In the consent order, the Michigan State Medical Society was no longer allowed to coerce third-party payors into accepting the cost-containment terms it dictated.

Finally, in a private antitrust action, *Kartell* v. *Blue Shield of Massachusetts, Inc.* [749 F. 2d 922 (1984)], Blue Shield, which enrolled more than 50 percent of the Massachusetts population, was sued by Kartell, a physician, on behalf of fellow physicians, because of Blue Shield's stringent reimbursement policies. Blue Shield would not allow physicians to increase their revenues by charging their patients a fee in addition to the fee paid by Blue Shield. The Court of Appeals found that Blue Shield was not in violation of the Sherman Act and should be able to pay what it considered to be a market price for physician services in order to compete. That is, Blue Shield was exercising its right as a cost-conscious buyer.

This group of cases from the demand side illustrates how antitrust policy can alter the demand for health care. Since insurance coverage usually means an increased demand for health care (the demand curve is shifted upward to the right), a cost-conscious buyer may be able to shift the demand curve to the left. This downward shift in the demand curve may reduce the potential increase in utilization occasioned by the presence of insurance.

Antitrust and an Increase in Supply

AMA v. U.S. [317 US 519 (1943)] involved an attempt by physicians to curtail the entry of a health maintenance organization, Group Health Association, into the Washington, D.C., area. Physicians who elected to work for Group Health Association were denied hospital staff privileges, isolated from the medical society, and subjected to verbal abuse and peer pressure from area physicians. The Supreme Court found that the American Medical Association and the local medical society were guilty of concerted criminal action in violation of Section 1 of the Sherman Act and ordered them to cease coercing physicians who wanted to work for Group Health Association. By the mid-1990s, Group Health Association (now Insurance Group Health Plan) had more than 100,000 members—members who would have been denied their choice of HMO membership if the local medical society and the American Medical Association had prevailed five decades earlier.

The Goldfarb decision, which subjected the learned professions to the antitrust laws, ushered in the current generation of antitrust litigation. An important objective of *Federal Trade Commission v. American Medical Association* [94 FTC 701 (1979), aff'd. 638 F. 2d 443 (2d Cir. 1980), aff'd. 452 US 960 (1982)], one of the first cases brought after Goldfarb, was to attempt to increase the supply of information in the marketplace. Economists have always considered information to be an essential good, or commodity, in the marketplace. In health care, as in other sectors providing goods and services, consumers or managed care plans with an increased supply of information can reduce costs by searching for the particular price or quality of service they desire; in effect, information creates more competition as the providers compete on the basis of price and quality.

In *Federal Trade Commission v. American Medical Association*, it was alleged that the American Medical Association inhibited the supply of information from physicians by making various forms of information dissemination a violation of the AMA code of ethics, which prohibited the solicitation of patients. (The American Dental Association had a similar prohibition on advertising by dentists.) In May 1982, the Supreme Court affirmed the Court of Appeals ruling that the American Medical Association violated Section 5 of the Federal Trade Commission Act.

Supply of Managed Care Firms

In the same suit against the American Medical Association, the FTC alleged that the AMA inhibited the growth of contract practice medicine, an arrangement that enabled a group of physicians to contract with a private payor of health services, such as a preferred provider organization or a health maintenance organization, which would then compete against physicians who were not members of the group. After the Supreme Court decision, the AMA code of ethics could no longer prohibit contract medicine.

A number of federal antitrust actions have prevented physicians from hindering the growth of health maintenance organizations. The growth of health maintenance organizations is consistent with a competitive framework for a number of reasons. First, health maintenance organizations are additional competitors in the marketplace, increasing the scope of consumer choice. Second, health maintenance organizations may engender competition in the fee-for-service sector, which may put downward pressure on hospitalization rates in that sector.

Two early antitrust cases involved physicians in fee-for-service medicine who interfered with HMO growth. The first, *FTC* v. *Medical Service Corporation of Spokane County* [88 FTC 906 (1976)], involved an FTC complaint against the Medical Service Corporation, a Blue Shield plan, for interfering with the growth of HMOs in the eastern portion of the state of Washington. Physicians were not allowed to become participating members of the state's Blue Shield plan if they worked for an HMO. Since the Blue Shield plan was the largest insurer in its region, this was a significant sanction against HMO physicians. In a consent order, Medical Service Corporation of Spokane County agreed not to discriminate against HMO-based physicians.

In a closely related case, *FTC* v. *Forbes Health System Medical Staff* [94 FTC 1042 (1979)], the Federal Trade Commission filed suit against the Forbes Health System medical staff in Pittsburgh, which prevented physicians affiliated with HMOs from obtaining hospital staff privileges. Without access to hospitals, many physicians could not practice medicine. In the consent order, the Forbes Health System physicians had to refrain from discriminating against physicians who elected to join HMOs.

The effect of both these cases was to allow HMOs to compete in the marketplace based on their own merits. The Federal Trade Commission did not endorse HMOs; rather, it provided the opportunity for consumers to choose among health plans.

Courts have not always ruled in favor of competition or the consumer in cases involving the formation of health maintenance organizations or preferred provider organizations. For instance, in *Arizona* v. *Maricopa County Medical Society* [457 US 332 (1982)], the United States Supreme Court ruled in a 4–3 decision that the Maricopa Foundation for Medical Care, a nonprofit Arizona corporation, had violated Section 1 of the Sherman Act by engaging in the fixing of maximum prices. Approximately 1,750 physicians, or 70 percent of the county's private physicians, belonged to the Maricopa Foundation. Each of the physicians agreed to a maximum fee for his or her services. In addition, the foundation reviewed physician treatments for medical necessity. Physicians' diagnoses and prescribed lengths of stay were reviewed prior to the admission of their patients to hospitals.

A 70-percent market share by a single entity in a marketplace might be of antitrust concern because of the potential for the abuse of market power. However, a significant market share is only harmful when there are barriers to entry into the marketplace. If new firms can enter the market, monopoly profits earned by the firm with the large market share can be dissipated. In *Maricopa*, there did not appear to be barriers to health maintenance organizations entering the Arizona market. Market shares of HMOs in Arizona and in Phoenix (the center of Maricopa County) grew dramatically just prior to the antitrust suit. In addition, there were a large number of commercial insurers in the market.

The Supreme Court ruled that the Maricopa Foundation was illegal because of its price-fixing activities. Price fixing per se had been found to be illegal in a series of earlier Supreme Court decisions, but the Maricopa case involved maximum-price fixing. Physicians could set prices lower than the maximum if the demand for their services warranted a lower price. The Maricopa Foundation may have been a procompetitive force in the marketplace, especially when it competed with other fee-for-service plans.

Supply of Nonphysician Providers

Some physicians have attempted to limit competition from allied health professionals. In *Wilk* v. *American Medical Association* [895 F. 2d 352 (1990)], for example, the American Medical Association, a number of specialty medical associations, and a number of physicians were accused of refusing to deal professionally with chiropractors and of questioning chiropractors' ability to perform certain services. In addition, some physician groups refused to accept referrals from chiropractors or would deny chiropractors access to hospital staffs and hospital diagnostic services. The Seventh Circuit Court found the American Medical Association to be in violation of Section 1 of the Sherman Act.

In *Weiss* v. *York* [745 F. 2d 786 (1984)], osteopathic physicians in York, Pennsylvania, brought suit against York Hospital for violating Sherman Act Sections 1 and 2 by discriminating against osteopathic physicians in awarding staff privileges. The court's decision in favor of the plaintiff was based, in part, on the fact that an entire class of providers was discriminated against. Moreover, the court believed that osteopaths, if allowed hospital staff privileges, would generate significant competition for physicians.

In both suits, the courts ruled in favor of the plaintiff. In the same way antitrust rulings improved the variety and number of managed care plans, these rulings improved the variety and number of allied health professionals.

Supply of Physicians

One way physicians exclude competitors is to impose restrictions on staff privileges at hospitals. Physicians and the hospitals with which they are associated may believe that they can limit competition from other physicians and hospitals if they can be influential in selecting their own prospective colleagues.

In *Robinson* v. *Magovern* [521 F. Supp. 842 (1981), aff'd. mem. 688 F. 2d 824 3d Cir. (1982)], cardiac surgeon Robinson was denied privileges on the staff of Allegheny General Hospital because surgeon Magovern and the other physicians on the staff of the hospital believed that Robinson had neither the interest in research nor the personality to be acceptable to the hospital. The executive committee and Allegheny General Hospital argued that Robinson would not be acceptable to the hospital because he would not concentrate all of his practice at Allegheny General and might not be able to "function harmoniously with the medical staff, the residents, and the support personnel" [521 F. Supp. 875].

The court ruled that a hospital must be able to select the surgeons with whom it can best compete in the marketplace. Moreover, according to the court, Allegheny General Hospital does not have a monopoly in the relevant Pittsburgh areas. If the hospital, to the benefit of its existing staff, were to raise its prices much above other hospitals, patients and insurers might increasingly use other hospitals in Pittsburgh. Moreover, the confirmation of Allegheny's prerogative of refusing privileges to Robinson suggests that hospitals and staff physicians can continue to compete on the basis of their perception of a quality-oriented medical staff.

In *Jefferson Parish Hospital* v. *Hyde* [466 US 2 (1984)], the hospital had an exclusive contract with its staff anesthesiologists. A prospective staff anesthesiologist, Hyde, sued the hospital, suggesting that exclusive contracts are anticompetitive. In addition, Hyde complained that an anticompetitive tie-in arrangement existed between the hospital and the anesthesiologists so that a patient who had surgery at the hospital had no choice but to use the hospital's anesthesiologists. The court suggested, however, that the hospital did not have monopoly power since it was competing against other hospitals in the area. Moreover, if the physicians under the exclusive contract attempted to capture additional profits, they could be replaced at the expiration of their contract by a new group of physicians. As in *Robinson* v. *Magovern*, the court ruled that a hospital's right to determine the physicians with which it contracts in a competitive marketplace outweighs any potential restrictions on competition.

Finally, *Patrick* v. *Burget* [486 US 94 (1988)] reveals most vividly the potential conflict between the interests of physicians in determining the staff of the hospital with which they are associated and society's interest in maintaining or increasing the number of competitors. In Astoria, Oregon, a physician, Patrick, was denied referrals and dismissed from the city's only hospital, Columbia Memorial Hospital, because of practicing poor-quality care, according to physicians on the hospital's quality review committee. Patrick denied these claims, suggesting that he was dismissed because he had set up his own surgical practice, which competed directly with the Astoria Clinic staffed by his colleagues at the hospital who had conspired to eliminate him as a competitor. Although the defendants had won in the Court of Appeals, the Supreme Court decided in Dr. Patrick's favor, suggesting that peer review committees that examine quality are not automatically immune from antitrust litigation.

In *Patrick* v. *Burget*, the quality of physician care was determined for all the physicians in Astoria by the hospital's quality review committee. There was little choice for the community but to abide by the judgment of the reviewing physicians in their definition of quality. A particularly strong case would have had to be made that the proficiency of a competing physician was clearly inferior, since a competitor would have been eliminated from the only hospital in the city. After the *Patrick* v. *Burget* decision, hospital peer review committees were not absolutely immune from antitrust litigation by physicians who might be excluded from the marketplace.

Supply of Nonhospital and Hospital Providers

In a case involving competition between a hospital and an urgent care center, physicians on the staff of John C. Lincoln Hospital and Health Center thwarted an attempt by Lincoln to open an out-patient urgent care center within three miles of the hospital. Physicians on the hospital staff were concerned that the urgent care center might result in lower costs, creating additional competition for the physicians and the hospital. The Federal Trade Commission brought suit against the physicians, which resulted in a consent agreement in which the physicians agreed not to coerce, threaten, or boycott Lincoln Hospital [*FTC* v. *Medical Staff of John G. Lincoln Hospital and Health Center*, 106 FTC 291 (1985)].

In 1979, American Medical International acquired a competing hospital, French Hospital, in San Luis Obispo, California. The Federal Trade Commission [107 FTC 310 (1984)] maintained that the acquisition violated Section 7 of the Clayton Act by eliminating a competitor from the marketplace and increasing the concentration of hospital services in San Luis Obispo and San Luis Obispo County. Both the full commission and the FTC administrative law judge agreed with the commission complaint. Subsequent to the decision, American Medical International had to sell the hospital to another purchaser.

In another hospital merger challenged by the Federal Trade Commission [106 FTC 361 (1985), aff'd. 807 F. 2d 1381 (7th Cir. 1986), cert. denied, 197 S. Ct. 1975 (1987)], Hospital Corporation of America purchased the Hospital Affiliates International chain of hospitals as well as the Health Care Corporation chain. The geographic market in which these chains owned or contract-managed hospitals was defined as the Chattanooga, Tennessee, area. Hospital Corporation of America was found to own or manage five of the eleven hospitals in the city and 26 percent of hospital services in what the court described as a highly concentrated market. The court found

Hospital Corporation of America to be in violation of Section 7 of the Clayton Act and ordered the company to divest itself of two hospitals and to terminate its management contract with a third hospital. By insisting upon divestiture of the two hospitals, the Federal Trade Commission returned the hospital market to its premerger status quo. No additional competitors were created. However, without FTC action, there would have been fewer firms in the market. This reduction in supply might have resulted in increases in prices to patients and third parties.

In *U.S. v. Rockford Memorial Corp.*, as Chapter 3 pointed out, the court concluded that the reduction of the number of hospitals would mean higher prices and a reduction in competition. The fact that both hospitals were nonprofit seemed to make little difference in the court's analysis. In view of the cost-conscious insurer in the 1990s and no discernible economies of scale, most economists would support the opinion in *U.S. v. Rockford Memorial Corp.* rather than the opinion in *U.S. v. Carillion Health System.*

Supply of Physician-Hospital Organizations

The number of physician-hospital organizations (PHOs) has increased in recent years. These organizations may be thought of as a form of vertical integration: physicians bring patients to the hospital, and the output or patient outcome becomes the result of a hospital in-patient or out-patient visit.

This form of vertical integration may have the benefits of reducing constant contracting costs between physicians and hospitals and may provide better communication of information between them. When a hospital has monopoly power, however, it may be used to discipline potential new physicians who would not be able to practice medicine without hospital staff privileges.

U.S. v. Health Choice of Northwest Missouri, Inc., Heartland Health System, Inc., and St. Joseph Physicians, Inc. (complaint filed 1995)

In *St. Joseph*, it was alleged by the U.S. Department of Justice that the Heartland Health System, Inc., which operated the only hospital in St. Joseph, Missouri, had colluded with St. Joseph Physicians, Inc. (SJPI), to keep managed care plans out of the area. It was alleged that 85 percent of the 130 physicians in the county owned shares of SJPI. Moreover, Heartland and SJPI formed their own managed care plan, Health Choice, which consisted mostly of SJPI physicians on their staff. After the formation of Health Choice, there were no new managed care plans which had entered the St. Joseph market.

The combination of nearly all physicians and a monopoly hospital can be strong enough to deter entry of a managed care plan. A new managed care plan would find it difficult to enter the market place without negotiating and contracting with physicians in the marketplace. Both the existing physicians and the existing hospital had incentives to prevent managed care plans from entering the marketplace as well as to prevent the entry of physicians who might be potential competitors. Thus, it is not surprising, with potential entrants kept out of the market, that the existing physicians in the Heartland Health System began collectively to set the fees they would charge.

St. Joseph's was resolved with a consent agreement with the Department of Justice. SJPI would no longer be able to dictate the managed care plans with which physicians could sign contracts. Health Choice was also enjoined from selecting physicians only through SJPI.

U.S. and State of Connecticut v. HealthCare Partners, Inc., Danbury Area IPA, Inc., and Danbury Health Systems, Inc. (complaint filed September 1995)

In this complaint, the Department of Justice alleged that the Danbury Hospital, a purported monopoly, aligned itself with the Danbury Area Independent Practice Association (DAIPA). The owners of DAIPA were the active members of Danbury Hospital's medical staff, and membership in DAIPA was open only to doctors on the hospital's medical staff. More than 98 percent of the medical staff at Danbury Hospital had affiliated with DAIPA. Both the Danbury Hospital and DAIPA had an equal controlling interest in HealthCare Partners, Inc., which served as a joint negotiating entity with managed care firms that wished to enter the market. The Danbury Hospital would contract only with HealthCare Partners and would not negotiate with any other managed care plan. Control over hospital admitting privileges made it nearly impossible for new physicians to enter the market. The complaint also asserted that HealthCare Partners had signed contracts with only two managed care plans. The complaint termed the fee schedules under these contracts to be "generous."

In the consent order negotiated with the Justice Department in February 1996, the defendants agreed to stop refusing to negotiate with any prospective payor who might enter the marketplace and to eliminate any incentives to deal exclusively with DAIPA or HealthCare Partners. The Danbury Hospital also had to stop denying staff privileges, without cause, to physicians who wanted to practice at the hospital. The aim of the consent order was to allow greater competition among physicians in Danbury as well as to remove barriers to entry to managed care plans.

Vertical Integration: Antitrust Perspective

Economists have suggested that vertical integration may have benefits for the organizations involved. One benefit is reduction in contract and transaction negotiation costs between and among firms. Thomas L. Greaney has suggested that vertical integration can also make it easier to pool capital, to spread financial risk, and to increase quality of care in the health care industry ["Managed Competition, Integrated Delivery Systems and Antitrust," *Cornell Law Review*, 79 (1994): 1507–1545, p. 1516]. However, vertical integration in physician-hospital organizations, for example, where one entity has monopoly power, can lead to an enhancement of monopoly power for both firms. In *St. Joseph* and *Danbury*, each of the hospitals had monopoly power. Because of the monopoly power of the hospitals, physicians could be excluded from staff privileges and the physician marketplace.

Antitrust in the Health Care Sector: Evaluation

The courts and the Federal Trade Commission appear to have ruled in favor of more, not less, competition in the health care sector. The rulings have favored nonphysician providers competing with physicians, physicians competing against one another, and more competition among hospitals. In cases involving staff privileges at hospitals, the courts, except in *Patrick* v. *Burget*, allowed existing staff arrangements to continue unless an entire class of providers was denied privileges. In each of the demand-side cases, the courts allowed the third party to attempt to contain costs and ruled against physician or dentist boycotts of third-party payors.

The courts appear to have applied the antitrust laws in health care as they would have applied them in any other sector, assuming that competition rather than planning or regulation would curb excessive costs and improve quality. Those who believe that the health care sector is different from other sectors might disagree with these attempts to make health care industries more competitive. However, each industry is unique, and antitrust would be irrelevant if each industry were to attempt to secure an exemption from litigation on the grounds that its industry was somehow different from other industries in the economy.

Antitrust appears to be as important to a competitive policy in health care as it is to a competitive policy in any other sector. A competitive policy can make an industry more efficient, and in health care, absent any rightward shift in demand, it can contribute to a reduction in costs. Without antitrust, it would not be difficult to imagine health care dominated by the higher-priced physicians (without the choice of lower-priced nonphysician providers) and without any controls on prices and costs by third-party payors. One might also predict a larger number of horizontal mergers, which would increase concentration.

The health care marketplace as a whole has become more competitive since the Goldfarb decision in 1975. There has been substantial growth in a variety of managed care plans, growth that might have been slowed considerably if physicians had been allowed to interfere. Antitrust may also have improved access to care because of a greater number of providers in the marketplace. Moreover, antitrust may have had deterrent effects on anticompetitive behavior: litigation costs in antitrust cases can be substantial, and firms found in violation of the Sherman Act may be fined an amount equal to three times the damages of the antitrust action.

Is antitrust a public or private good? That is, to what extent should the government rather than the private sector bring antitrust cases that reduce competition? [Warren Greenberg, "Private Antitrust as a Public Good," *Loyola Consumer Law Reporter*, 8 (1995–1996): 118–124]. More than 90 percent of all antitrust cases are currently brought by firms in the private sector; the Marshifield Clinic case is the foremost example. The cost to Blue Cross and Blue Shield of Wisconsin, the largest insuring organization in the state, of the antitrust action against the 500-physician-member Marshfield clinic will be at least $3 million. Private antitrust cases might be brought when a firm such as Blue Cross and Blue Shield of Wisconsin has a substantial market share so that it may capture most of the awarded damages if it wins the case. Firms may also bring cases when there is a potential time lag before new entrants, such as new insuring organizations, realize the benefits of increased competition without bearing the costs of litigation. Finally, it has been shown that the equity value of an average plaintiff had gained 1.2 percent when an antitrust suit is announced [John M. Bizjak and Jeffrey L. Coles, "The Effect of Private Antitrust Litigation on the Stock-Market Valuation of the Firm," *American Economic Review*, 85 (1995): 436–462].

Without these conditions, public sector antitrust suits might be brought where there are innovative legal theories to be tested and when potential private plaintiff firms have market shares low enough that most of the benefits of a successful antitrust suit accrue to other parties. In addition, public antitrust suits might be brought when, because of a hospital merger or collusion among hospitals, for example, the remaining hospitals could set their prices under the umbrella of the merged hospital.

In the future, antitrust litigation may play an even larger role in the health care sector. An increasing number of physicians graduating from medical school, an increasing number of excess beds, and an increasing aggressiveness among nonphysician providers—within tightened private- and public-sector budgets—all point to increased antitrust activity as providers compete for a shrinking per capita reimbursement.

Health Care Marketplace

In 1994, in a private antitrust action, Blue Cross and Blue Shield of Wisconsin, the largest insurer in Wisconsin, and its HMO, Compcare, brought suit against the fifth-largest group of physicians in the United States, the Marshfield Clinic, and its HMO, Security Health Plan, Inc. The Marshfield Clinic is of interest because of the size and depth of its vertical integration in health care services.

In northwestern Wisconsin, home of the Marshfield Clinic, 300 Marshfield Clinic physicians, mostly specialists, practiced medicine. In addition, approximately 100 physicians, mostly family physicians, practiced medicine in 23 clinics scattered throughout rural northwestern Wisconsin. In 9 of 13 clinics, Marshfield Clinic family physicians had more than 60 percent of the patient market, and in 8 of the 13 clinics, Marshfield Clinic pediatricians had more than 60 percent of the patient market (data were reliably reported for only these 13 clinics).

The Marshfield Clinic physicians were closely linked with the 524-bed St. Joseph's Hospital in Marshfield. St. Joseph's Hospital was the largest hospital in northwestern Wisconsin, as well as the area's most technologically advanced hospital. It was the only hospital of the four hospitals in the relevant geographic market that performed sophisticated open-heart surgery, neonatology, and oncology procedures. In addition, Wisconsin state certificate-of-need laws made it difficult for new hospitals to enter the area or for any hospital to purchase the technologically advanced equipment. Only Marshfield Clinic physicians were allowed staff privileges at St. Joseph's. In fourteen specialty markets, such as coronary bypass surgery, Marshfield Clinic physicians had more than 60 percent of the patient market.

The Marshfield Clinic physicians had begun an IPA-model HMO, Security Health Plan of Wisconsin, Inc., which, in 1992, had 70,000 members. Marshfield Clinic primary care and physician specialists participated in Security Health Plan along with more than 300 independent physicians who were not associated with the Marshfield Clinic. Physicians who participated in Security Health Plan were required to refer patients to Marshfield Clinic specialists and St. Joseph's Hospital. It was also expected that the non-Marshfield Clinic physicians would refer their patients who were not members of Security Health Plan to the Marshfield Clinic.

Blue Cross and Blue Shield asserted in their complaint that they could not launch their HMO, CompCare, in northwestern Wisconsin because Marshfield Clinic physicians would not participate or negotiate with them. Moreover, the high market shares of Marshfield Clinic physicians were asserted to have led to higher physician fees. The charges in *Marshfield*, therefore, were not dissimilar to those in *St. Joseph* and *Danbury*.

Although the U.S. District Court in Wisconsin agreed with all the elements of the Blue Cross and Blue Shield complaint, the U.S. Court of Appeals reversed the lower court's decision. The higher court mistakenly focused on the "correct" definition of the HMO product market rather than on Marshfield Clinic monopolization of physician services or the foreclosure of the formation of managed care plans in the health care financing market. The Court of Appeals correctly believed that the plaintiff's emphasis on the HMO as the relevant market was too narrow, and that cross-elasticities of demand and supply dictated that the product market should include all health care financing mechanisms.

Chapter 8 Appendix

Blue Cross & Blue Shield United of Wisconsin, CompCare Health Services Insurance Corporation, Appellants
v.
Marshfield Clinic and Security Health Plan of Wisconsin, Inc., Appellees

Nos. 95-1965, 95-2140
U.S. Court of Appeals, Seventh Circuit
Decided September 18, 1995

Although Marshfield is a town of only 20,000 people in a largely rural region, the Marshfield Clinic is the fifth largest physician-owned Clinic in North America, with annual revenues in excess of $200 million. The Clinic has its main office in Marshfield but it has 21 branch offices scattered throughout the 14 counties of north central Wisconsin (p. 1409).

It is true that because of the sparsity of the physician population in north central Wisconsin the physicians employed by the Clinic have a large share of the market for physician services, since, for a primary care anyway (an important qualification—people will go a long way for a liver transplant), that market is a local one.... CompCare is unable to show that in what it chooses to regard as the relevant geographic market or series of linked geographic markets for physician services the Marshfield Clinic employed 50 percent or more of the physicians serving the market (p. 1411).

CompCare is able to derive larger shares only by defining submarkets of specific, very narrowly defined medical procedures, called "Diagnostic Related Groups" (p. 1411).

The Clinic is said to have agreed with some of its competitors, in particular the North Central Health Protection Plan, an HMO that had 37,000 subscribers, to divide markets, a practice that violates section 1 of the Sherman Act (p. 1415).

We think the evidence of a division of markets, though a little scanty, was sufficient to sustain the jury's verdict on this (and only this) aspect of the case (p. 1416).

9
Regulation and Competition in Health Care

In nearly all industries, the goverment has been or is a regulatory presence. Regulation of electric utility rates, size of agricultural output, tariffs and quotas on imported goods and services, and licensing of taxicabs are just a few of the many government regulations in the American economy. Government regulation also pervades the health care sector.

Government Regulation of Industries Other than Health Care

Government regulation takes several forms, one of which is regulation of price. In 1887, for example, the Interstate Commerce Commission began establishing the minimum railroad charges for interstate freight shipments. Price regulation was extended to common carrier trucking, water carriers, and pipelines, before gradual deregulation of prices in the 1980's [N. A. Glaskowsky, *Effects of Deregulation on Motor Carriers* (Westport CT: Eno Foundation of Transportation, 1986)].

Regulation of prices occurs outside the transportation sector. Even the price of money (the interest rate) for time and savings accounts was regulated by the Board of Governors of the Federal Reserve System and the Federal Deposit Insurance Corporation so that rates would not exceed a predetermined level. In 1980, the Depository Institutions Deregulation and Monetary Control Act eliminated the artificially imposed interest rate ceilings on these deposit accounts [K. Cooper and D. R. Fraser, *Banking Deregulation and the New Competition in Financial Services* (Cambridge, MA: Ballinger, 1984)].

Regulation also directly affects the prices of natural gas, water, and electric power utilities. A utility experiences a decline in its long-run average costs per unit as it produces additional units, due to the high fixed costs of the capital investment of the firm. These economies of scale may allow only one firm to survive in the industry as a natural monopoly, since it can reduce prices below those of any potential entrants. As a monopoly, the firm would be able to charge a monopoly price. To prevent the firm from realizing a supracompetitive rate of return from a monopoly price, prices are set equal to the average costs of the firm.

In addition to regulations that affect price directly, other regulations affect price indirectly. Government regulation of "surplus" agricultural production has created artificially high prices for farm products such as wheat, corn, and tobacco with low elasticities of demand. If the market price falls, farmers can receive government subsidies up to a predetermined target price. [Erik Lichtenberg and David Zilberman, "The Welfare Economics of Price Supports in U.S. Agriculture," *American Economic Review*, 76 (1986): 1135–1141].

Government regulation may limit new competition or create barriers to entry into industries. The regulation of imports (import quotas) and the imposition of tariffs (taxes on foreign commodities) hamper competition from foreign firms and raises prices. The Civil Aeronautics Board, in addition to discouraging price competition among airlines, regulated entry of new carriers to the extent that not a single new trunk line entered the airline services market from the creation of the board in 1938 until its gradual abolishment beginning in 1978 [Steven Morrison and Clifford Winston, *The Economic Effects of Airline Deregulation* (Washington, DC: Brookings Institute, 1986)].

Economists have suggested that the prices set by regulatory authorities are not socially optimal because it is unlikely that the government is able to compute the marginal costs and marginal revenue of each individual firm or set of firms in order to set economically efficient prices. Moreover, the government, with its actions on demand and supply, may create artificially high prices and high profits. Likewise, government entry restrictions result in higher profits than if the industries were more competitive. Regulations that restrict output of the existing firms in an industry also attempt to ensure that prices and profits are higher than they are at the competitive level.

Safety regulations imposed on firms also affect price. For example, the Federal Aviation Administration requires certain standards of safety on airplanes. By requiring seat belts, qualification standards for pilots, and standards of construction and maintenance on airplanes, regulations directly affect costs and indirectly affect price. Mandatory air-bag installation for front-seat passengers for model year 1998 will also have the effect of increasing the price of automobiles as well as, paradoxically, increasing more aggressive driving [Steven Peterson et al., "Are Drivers of Air-Bagged Cars More Aggressive? A Test of the Offsetting Behavior Hypothesis," *Journal of Law and Economics*, 38 (1995): 251–264]. Individuals may also use fewer safety precautions if they believe that products are safer. Viscusi and Cavallo found that mandated child safety devices on cigarette lighters, which may cause increases in prices, relieved parents from taking some precautionary steps toward children's access to lighters. However, the authors found that the safety devices did outweigh any diminished precautionary efforts [W. Kip Viscusi and Gerald O. Cavallo, "The Effect of Product Safety Regulation on Safety Precautions," *Risk Analysis*, 14, (1994): 917–930].

The Federal Trade Commission (FTC.) prohibits false, misleading, and deceptive advertising. This may result in lower costs to consumers if consumers are able to rely on the information of sellers without having to bear the transactions costs of increased search [Raymond D. Sauer and Keith B. Leffler, "Did the Federal Trade Commission's Advertising Substantiation Program Promote More Credible Advertising?" *American Economic Review*, 80 (1990): 191–203]. Sauer and Leffler found that the FTC's requirement that advertising claims must have prior, full documentation and adequate substantiation resulted in more credible, verifiable advertising. In contrast, Sam Peltzman found that the effects of FTC regulation are unclear for consumers, although actions brought by the FTC can negatively affect the capital value of firms ["The Effects of FTC Advertising Regulation," *Journal of Law and Economics*, 24 (1981): 403–448].

Firms that pollute the environment create externalities, or costs the public as a whole must bear. To offset the external costs of pollution, the government may require that firms install pollution controls or pay pollution taxes. If firms have relatively inelastic demand curves, the increased costs of pollution controls and taxes may be passed on to customers in the form of higher prices. Recently, however, the Environmental Protection Agency (EPA) began to assess the costs of cleaning hazardous wastes and other sorts of pollution versus the benefits of a cleaner environment [W. Kip Viscusi, "Economic Foundations of the Current Regulatory Reform Efforts," *Journal of Economic Perspectives*, 10 (Summer 1996): 119–134, p. 120]. Moreover, EPA emissions regulations have also experimented with a least-cost approach to regulation that solicits bids from private firms in a competitive environment for permits to clean up pollution [pp. 128–129].

Some economists suggest that regulation may stem from the demand for regulation in the political marketplace, regardless of imperfections in the economic marketplace. That is, industries may be regulated because firms in the industry desire to have the protection of government regulation to curb competitive pressures from inside or outside the industry [George J. Stigler, "The Theory of Economic Regulation," *Bell Journal of Economics and Management Science*, 2 (1971): 3–21]; [Sam Peltzman; "Toward a More General Theory of Regulation," *The Journal of Law and Economics* 19 (1976): 211–240]. Regulated prices, restricted entry, and limited production are usually in the interest of existing firms in order to gain higher profits. Furthermore, existing firms may have considerable political influence over government legislation and the regulatory process [Stigler, 1971; Peltzman, 1976]. The agricultural industry has been most outspoken in demanding governmental restrictions on its output, automobile manufacturers have demanded restrictions on the import of foreign automobiles, and the trucking industry has supported rate regulation.

Regulation in the Health Care Sector

What are the types of regulation in health care and what are the effects of the regulation? Similar to other industries, regulations in the health care industry restrict entry, raise prices, and limit output. In addition, health insurance firms receive special regulatory attention. Regulations have also been enacted to attempt to improve quality and safety in health care goods and services.

Regulations That Restrict Entry into Provider Markets

A number of regulations restrict entry into the hospital, physician, managed care, and nursing home markets. In 1910, the so-called Flexner Report, written by educator Abraham Flexner and the Carnegie Foundation for the Advancement of Teaching, recommended a reduction in the number of medical schools and medical students in order to improve the quality of medical care. The American Medical Association used this report as justification to limit the number of medical school graduates [Reuben Kessel, "Price Discrimination in Medicine," *Journal of Law and Economics*, 1 (1958): 20–53]. Since the states had designated the AMA as the accreditor of medical schools, the AMA was able to decertify medical schools while ostensibly increasing the quality of care. Between 1906 and 1944, it closed 93 medical schools [Kessel, 1958]. As described in Chapter 2, the AMA placed further restrictions on paramedicals and managed care systems.

State certificate-of-need laws, enacted in the mid-1970s, regulated the number of hospital beds, the dollar value of hospital equipment, and the number of nursing homes. Proponents of certificate-of-need laws believed that an increase in the number of hospital beds would increase costs, since empty beds would likely be filled. Moreover, hospitals appeared to compete by purchasing new technologies to attract physicians who, in turn, would admit patients. If there were a limit to the acquisition of new technology, the total costs of new technology by all hospitals would be smaller. Certificate-of-need laws, however, may serve to protect the interests of existing hospitals by limiting the expansion of competitors or entry of new hospitals.

Many states, in legislation opposed by many hospitals, have now abandoned certificate-of-need laws because studies revealed that certificate of need did little to reduce total hospital investment. In states where certificate-of-need laws appeared to limit the growth of new beds, hospitals increased their investment in new facilities and equipment [David C.

Salkever and Thomas W. Bice, "The Impact of Certificate-of-Need Controls on Hospital Investment," *Milbank Memorial Fund Quarterly*, 54 (1976): 195–214]. Paul L. Joskow ["Alternative Regulatory Mechanisms for Controlling Hospital Costs," in *A New Approach to the Economics of Health Care*, ed. M. Olson (Washington, DC: American Enterprise Institute, 1981), pp. 219–257] also found that certificate-of-need regulation had no effect on either the level or the rate of growth of hospital expenditures.

Historically, state "freedom-of-choice" laws specified that groups of physicians or groups of hospitals could not be formed by employers, insuring organizations, or any other groups to compete against the remaining physicians or hospitals in the state. Until the freedom-of-choice laws were repealed in the early 1980s, preferred provider organizations and some staff-model health maintenance organizations could not be established because all providers had to be offered in the health care plan [Charles D. Weller, "'Free Choice' as a Restraint of Trade in American Health Care Delivery and Insurance," *Iowa Law Review*, 69 (1984): 1351–1394]. However, with the increase in number of preferred provider organizations, health maintenance organizations, and managed care firms that limit or reduce payments to out-of-network providers, freedom-of-choice or "any willing provider" laws had again been enacted in forty states by 1995. States have applied these laws to providers of health care services, to pharmacies, to ancillary services such as medical laboratories, and to independent allied health professionals [George Washington University Intergovernmental Health Policy Project, *State Any Willing Provider Laws and Related Activities: Implications for Technology*, July 1995, pp. 1–5]. Any willing provider laws make it difficult for managed care plans to negotiate the best prices and quality with a given set of providers. Providers whose prices are too high or whose quality is unacceptable to the managed care plan cannot be deleted from a plan's list of providers. Thus, any willing provider laws increase costs for all patients.

Regulation of Price

Price regulation has been extensive in health care, perhaps more so than in any other industry, for a number of reasons. First, rapidly increasing costs in health care may have affected the amount of regulation. State governments paying an increasing amount for health services (primarily Medicaid) have, of course, less money available for other state programs and therefore face increasing pressures to reduce health care expenditures [Philip Fanara, Jr., and Warren Greenberg, "Factors Affecting the Adoption of Prospective Reimbursement Programs by State Governments," in *Incentives v. Controls in Health Policy*, ed. Jack A. Meyer (Washington, DC: American Enterprise Institute, 1985), pp. 144–156]. The reasons behind President Nixon's 1971 Economic Stabilization Program (ESP), which regulated wages and prices in the health care sector as well as the rest of the economy, behind President Carter's 1979 proposed controls of hospital revenues, and behind Medicare's hospital (DRG) and physician payment (RBRVS) regulations were to curb increases in health care spending. The enactment of the RBRVS regulation of physician fees may have also been due to the government's desire to increase the relatively low fees of primary care physicians and reduce the relatively high fees of specialists.

In addition to the RBRVS price regulation of physicians and the DRG price regulation of hospitals discussed in Chapters 2 and 6, the states have instituted a number of prospective price controls on hospitals. In 1977, nine states utilized mandatory prospective reimbursement systems [Fanara and Greenberg]. Gerard F. Anderson suggests that a hoped for reduction of cost shifting to some private insurers may have also been a reason for the enactment of an all-payer system ["All-Payer Ratesetting: Down but Not Out," *Health Care Financing Review*, Annual Supplement, 1991, pp. 35–41]. It appears, however, that financial difficulties of the hospitals in Maryland were instrumental in their support of a rate setting commission.

The state of Maryland introduced all-payer rate setting on a hospital-by-hospital basis in 1971, and as of 1997, Maryland was the only state that regulated hospital rates. Selective contracting is not allowed in Maryland. All insurers, including Medicare, Medicaid, and managed care plans, must pay the same rates. The rates are paid for each unit of service. Direct and indirect costs are considered. Inflation and adjustments for increases in volume can alter future rates.

Hospitals in Maryland resemble firms under cartel theory. Because of certificate-of-need laws [George Washington University Intergovernmental Health Policy Project, *Fifty State Profiles: Health Care Reform, 1995*, October 1995, Table 4, pp. 9–10], entry and expansion of hospitals into the hospital market is difficult. Hospitals are forbidden to reduce rates or prices to any managed care plan or insurer. Each hospital is assured of surviving because the established rates cover all costs. Because of the state regulation, hospitals are exempt from state and federal antitrust laws [U.S. General Accounting Office, *Antitrust Enforcement Under Maryland's Hospital All-Payer System*, April 1994].

In view of the managed care cost-containment efforts shown in Chapter 3, it is surprising that the State of Maryland has continued with hospital rate regulation. Clearly, creating equity among buyers by eliminating cost shifting is inefficient if one insuring organization is stronger than another and can achieve lower prices for the firm and for its enrollees. Guarding hospitals against uncompensated care may be a goal of an all-payer system, but the problems of uncompensated care and the uninsured would be more efficiently addressed if tackled directly (see Chapter 11).

Joskow [1981], in his examination of the mandatory state prospective reimbursement programs, found "a significant reduction in the rate of growth of hospital expenditures [p. 255]." He cautioned, however, that many of the states that had introduced cost containment were high-cost states and perhaps the states in which costs could be curbed most readily. Frank A. Sloan ["Rate Regulation as a Strategy for Cost Control: Evidence from the Last Decade," *Milbank Memorial Fund Quarterly*, 61 (1983): 195–217] examined the effects of state regulatory programs on hospital costs. In general, he found very little effect in initial years but a substantial effect in reducing cost per admission thereafter. Sloan attributed the delay to the increase in regulatory expertise the government gained after the first years of cost containment. However, one might also expect that the regulated hospitals would, after a learning period, gain insights into the most effective ways to avoid cost containment and therefore escape the regulatory umbrella. Jack Hadley and Katherine Swartz also found that state regulatory programs, as well as Medicare's prospective payment system, had controlled increases in hospital costs between 1980 and 1984, although this decrease might have stemmed from a one-time drop because of the Prospective Payment System (PPS) or DRG system of Medicare regulation, reduction in quality of care, or gains in hospital efficiency ["The Impact on Hospital Costs Between 1980 and 1984 of Hospital Rate Regulation, Competition, and Changes in Health Insurance Coverage," *Inquiry*, 26 (1989): 35–47)].

Two recent studies, however, have suggested that hospital rate regulation has no effect on hospital costs. John J. Antel et al. ["State Regulation and Hospital Costs," *Review of Economics and Statistics*, 77 (1995): 416–422], in their cross-section analysis for the years 1968–1990, found that hospital rate regulation can reduce costs per day or per admission but has no effect on the more important variable of per capita hospital costs. Michael G. Vita finds that hospital rate-setting programs, looking at pooled cross-section time-series data between 1975 and 1985, had no effect on hospital expenditures ["The Impact of Hospital Rate Setting Programs on Hospital and Health Care Expenditures, 1975–1985", *Applied Economics*, 27 (1995): 917–923]. Moreover, he finds that rate-setting programs had no effect on the more important variable of *health care* expenditures. Since the Antel et al. and Vita studies are based on relatively early data, it is possible that rate regulation compared to the competitive environment of the late 1990s would fare worse.

Very few studies have examined the effects of price regulation on the quality of care, innovation, and market power of hospitals. Stephen Shortell and Edward F. X. Hughes ["The Effects of Regulation, Competition and Ownership on Mortality Rates Among Hospital Inpatients," *New England Journal of Medicine*, 318 (1988): 1100–1107] found a significant positive relationship between the stringency of state hospital rate-review programs (as well as the intensity of competition) and in-patient mortality rates for sixteen selected clinical conditions. Fewer resources may have been utilized for hospital patients, although, as the authors point out, mortality rates are not a complete measure of quality of care.

Insurance Regulation

The insurance industry is primarily regulated on a state-by-state basis. Since individuals purchase most insurance with the expectation that they will have coverage for at least a year, state governments have attempted to assure the solvency of insurance firms. Many states, therefore, regulate the level of insurance premiums to assure adequate assets and reserves. The regulations may reduce or eliminate bankruptcies, but they may also guarantee the survival of the least efficient insurance firms.

In many states, insurance firms are also required to offer certain benefits as part of the benefit package. Mandated benefits are usually outside the scope of hospital and physician benefits and might include, for example, a specified number of visits to psychologists or chiropractors. The effect of mandated benefits is to shift the demand curve for health services upward and to the right, which, at least initially, prompts an increase in price for these services. The effects of mandated benefits on employers might be equivalent to the effects of increases in the minimum wage [Lawrence H. Summers, "Some Simple Economics of Mandated Benefits," *American Economic Review*, 79 (1989): 177–183; Charles C. Brown, "Minimum Wage Laws: Are They Overrated?" *Journal of Economic Perspectives*, 2 (1988): 133–145]. Increases in minimum wages, according to Brown, may increase unemployment because of their positive effect on labor costs.

Blue Cross and Blue Shield plans have been regulated to a much greater extent than the commercial plans. Not only do many states regulate the Blues' premiums, but many states require the Blues to have open-enrollment periods for anyone willing to pay a regulated nongroup rate. Preexisting conditions, however, may not be covered by the Blues plans for at lease one year. The effects of regulating Blue Cross and Blue Shield are mixed. There is evidence that at least some Blues plans enroll a greater number (and a greater proportion) of high-risk individuals than do the commercial plans [Warren Greenberg, *Response to AIDS in the Private Sector* (Alexandria, VA: Capitol Publications, 1989)]. Fanara and Greenberg [1985] found, however, that the more competition Blue Cross and Blue Shield face from HMOs, the less likely they are to enroll high-risk individuals. It is not clear that an increase in the enrollment of high-risk individuals is sufficient to justify the exemption from health insurance premium, property, and income taxes that many Blue Cross and Blue Shield have enjoyed.

Reasons for Health Care Regulation

Regulation in health care is not due to economies of scale, which is the case in natural gas, electric, and water industries.

Government regulation of providers of health care also is not due to externalities like pollution or social costs. In contrast, government subsidizes scientific research, which may provide long-term health care benefits to society as a whole (social benefits). Government also immunizes children, at low cost, against contagious diseases that could affect society as a whole.

Safety regulation is as common in health care as in many complex industries. The Food and Drug Administration regulates pharmaceutical firms, requiring new drugs to undergo extensive tests until they are shown to be safe and effective for public use. However, the costs of developing more efficacious drugs have led to a decline in the number of new drugs brought to market as well as a large decline in drug research [Sam Peltzman, "An Evaluation of Consumer Protection Legislation: The 1962 Drug Amendments," *Journal of Political Economy*, 81 (1973): 1049–1091]. David Dranove also found that fewer drugs had been approved and that there are considerable delays in the approval process ["The Costs of Compliance with the 1962 FDA Amendments," *Journal of Health Economics*, 10 (1991): 235–238]. The 1984 Drug Amendments led to longer patent protection for existing drugs. In turn, the 1984 legislation made it easier for generics to be introduced into the marketplace. Studies of this legislation found greater entry of generic drugs but no diminution of price of established brands [Henry G. Grabowski and John M. Vernon, "Brand Loyalty, Entry, and Price Competition in Pharmaceuticals after the 1984 Drug Act," *Journal of Law and Economics*, 35 (1992): 331–350].

Health care deregulation has followed deregulation in other industries [Clifford Winston, "Economic Deregulation: Days of Reckoning for Microeconomists," *Journal of Economic Literature*, 31 (1993): 1263–1289]. Certificate-of-need laws and state regulation of hospital rates have been sharply reduced, and at the same time the number of managed care plans in both the public and private sectors has surged.

Competition in the Health Care Sector

What forms has competition taken in health care? Because of the presence of insurance, health care competition exists on two levels: competition among providers and competition among insuring organizations or managed care plans.

Competition Among Providers

Although insurance pays for two-thirds of health care expenditures, there is still competition among providers. Chapter 8 describes antitrust cases involving physicians who would not allow competing physicians staff privileges at hospitals. Evidence shows that some physicians relocate from areas with high physician-to-population ratios to less competitive rural areas [Al Williams et al., "How Many Miles to the Doctor?" *New England Journal of*

Medicine, 30 (1983): 958–963]. Mark V. Pauly ["Is Medical Care Different?" in *Competition in the Health Care Sector: Past, Present and Future*, ed. W. Greenberg (Germantown, MD: Aspen Publishers, 1978)] suggests that there is price-based competition among physicians such as pediatricians, whose services generally are not well covered by insurance.

Competition exists among hospitals and even between out-patient centers and hospitals. Chapter 8 describes the difficulties that some surgicenters may experience in delivering their services in areas that are near hospitals. There is a substantial amount of price and nonprice competition among hospitals. Hospitals, of course, have always competed by purchasing the most advanced forms of technological equipment. Evidence suggests that hospital markets encompass a larger geographic area and face a greater number of competitors than formerly recognized [Morrisey, Sloan, and Valvona, 1988].

Competition Among Insuring Organizations

Many economists believe that competition among insuring organizations or managed care plans may be the best avenue for improving the allocation of health care resources. Two of the most important factors in a competitive framework—factors not generally present when patients choose among providers—are found in competition among health insuring organizations. First, buyers of health plans (whether employers or individuals) are sensitive to prices of health insuring organizations since unlike hospital visits and tests, for example, purchases are not influenced by the presence of insurance. (To the extent that an employer pays the full cost of each plan that is offered, individuals, of course, are not sensitive). Second, buyers of health plans generally are well prepared to make informed choices in choosing a health plan. Advertising by health plans and information provided by employers can lead to a better evaluation of health plans by individuals. Individuals can speak with their firm's benefit counselors to secure additional information. Decisions need not be made immediately; employers usually provide a month in which to decide upon a plan. Moreover, the choice is not irrevocable; employees usually have the option of switching health plans at least once a year.

The employer often acts as a guarantor of quality for the health care plans it offers. The employer wants to retain employees, and one way to do so is to provide attractive health care benefits. If a health benefits plan does not conform to its promises, employees' allegiance to the employer may be reduced. In short, employers (even unions) in both the private and public sector may, as Alain C. Enthoven and Richard Kronick ["A Consumer-Choice Health Plan for the 1990's" (first of two parts), *New England Journal of Medicine*, 320 (1989): 29–37] suggest, act as sponsors in assisting employees to choose among plans.

Competition among health plans may be found in many employer groups in both the private and public sectors. As long as there is free entry into the market for health plans, premiums of health plans should be competitive. Even when choosing only a single plan to offer, an employer may take competitive bids from insuring organizations to get the plan with the best combination of premiums and benefits.

Enthoven's Consumer Choice Health Plan

Enthoven's consumer choice health plan is an important policy prescription for competition among health care plans. Enthoven makes a number of points in his proposal. First, he envisions competition among integrated financing and health care delivery systems, such as staff-model health maintenance organizations, with providers bearing most of the risk. According to Enthoven, traditional fee-for-service insurance firms will not be able to create incentives to achieve efficiency because providers are not at risk, although fee-for-service plans could continue to exist. An open-enrollment period would be held once a year. To assure maximum consumer choice under the Enthoven plan, employers in the private sector would not be able to contribute a greater amount to any single plan they offered. Although each plan would be community rated, individuals seeking a more expansive plan would have to pay a larger out-of-pocket contribution. There would be no overall cap on expenditures.

"Sponsors" would play a key role in providing information to enrollees. Sponsors might be employers, unions, state governments (which could have pools of high-risk individuals), and aggregate sponsors of the small firms that find it unprofitable to offer health insurance on their own to their employees. Sponsors would also assure standardized benefit packages among health plans. Each plan would be required to offer the same comprehensive benefits plan to all individuals; plans could not offer reduced benefit packages at lower prices to attract only healthy persons. Deductibles would not be allowed to exceed $250 per person [Alain C. Enthoven, *Theory and Practice of Managed Competition in Health Care Finance* (The Netherlands: Elsevier Science Publishing, 1988); Alain C. Enthoven and Richard Kronick, "A Consumer-Choice Health Plan for the 1990's," Parts 1 and 2, *New England Journal of Medicine*, 320 (1989): 29–37 and 94–101]. Indeed, insistence on competition among health plans without discrimination against high-risk individuals is an integral part of the Enthoven proposals.

Finally, sponsors would also guard against cream skimming and inequity in the health care system. Premiums would be adjusted based on age, gender, family composition, and retirement status [Alain C. Enthoven, "On the Ideal Market Structure for Third-Party Purchasing of Health Care," *Social Science and Medicine*, 39 (1994): 1413–1424, p. 1418]. In addition, payments would have to be made to each health plan by the sponsors for a few very costly chronic conditions [p. 1419]. Sponsors would have the continual responsibility of reviewing the payments as technology and treatment schemes evolve [p. 1419].

Competition among health plans, however, also entails potential complications. Variation would still remain within risk categories and it would be extremely difficult to eliminate cream skimming entirely. Risk selection would take place at the physician-patient level if physicians began to treat high-risk patients rudely. Health plans may also locate their offices in suburban areas where younger families may live. Although information might appear to be plentiful on the attributes of the plans, it would be imperfect information. Each plan has many dimensions, including its financial relationship with physicians, its quality of care, its cost-containment mechanisms, and its financial viability. If employees erred in their choice of health plan, they would find it difficult to change it before the next annual open-enrollment period.

Within this competitive framework (or indeed any framework in which individuals have insurance), individuals still have incentives to consume more health services than they would without health insurance. Individuals may consume services in which marginal benefits are nearly zero since there are no direct costs to the patient. Managed care firms may be able to curb some of these services with measures such as utilization review, but they must be cognizant of legal liability. In contrast, from society's viewpoint, the optimal allocation of all goods and services occurs when both benefits and costs are considered. The differences between an individual's incentives and the achievement of an optimal allocation of resources are discussed further in Chapter 10.

Clinton Health Care Reform Plan

In 1993, President Bill Clinton introduced a health care reform proposal, the Health Security Act ["A New Framework for Health Care," *New York Times*, November 14, 1993, p. 3]. The proposed Act called for managed competition and universal coverage, the two central components of the Enthoven plan. However, in a number of important respects it differed from the Enthoven plan and efficient health care markets in general.

There were four main economic entities in the Clinton proposal: individuals and businesses as ultimate purchasers of health care services, health care alliances as buying agents for individuals and businesses, health care plans (HMOs, fee-for-service plans, and other managed care organizations—termed accountable health plans), and the national health board. Small businesses and individuals would have been required to join the sole health alliance in a region so that the alliance could bargain with the health care plans to deliver quality and control costs. The health alliances would

Clinton Health Security Act

have been monopsonists in each region. If health plans already had strong incentives to bargain with providers, however, it was not clear what incremental value health care alliances between employer and health plan would have had in negotiating with providers [Warren Greenberg, "Monopsony Power and Managed Competition: Do Regional Alliances Make Sense?" *Journal of Subacute Care*, 1 (1994): 37–41]. Moreover, in the Clinton proposal, health alliances were to set fee schedules for fee-for-service physicians. Similar to one of the roles of the sponsors in the Enthoven plan, a report card on the quality of each health care plan would have been developed. *report cards*

Unlike the Enthoven plan, the Health Security Act contained a budget ceiling for each plan that was to be set by the national health board. Health care costs were not to exceed this cap, but how health care was to be rationed and at what level the ceiling would be set was not explained in the proposal. The national health board was also expected to limit increases in insurance premiums. Finally, to discourage discrimination against high-risk individuals, the national health board was to develop factors for risk adjustments for the accountable health plans as well as to update a standardized benefit package which would include comprehensive acute care coverage as well as some dental and mental health care benefits [Paul Starr and Walter A. Zelman, "A Bridge to Compromise: Competition under a Budget," *Health Affairs*, 12 (1993; supplement): 7–23].

Similar to the Enthoven plan, employer-based health insurance was to have been the mechanism by which individuals in the private sector would receive their health insurance. In the public sector, the Medicaid program was to be superseded by a program in which low-income individuals received federal assistance to purchase coverage through accountable health plans (AHPs). Medicare, however, would not have been altered.

The Clinton health care reform proposal attempted to use doses of competition, regulation, and outright rationing (with the use of budget ceilings) to achieve an efficient health care system, to control costs, and to provide universal coverage. A far-ranging proposal, it rested on the unsound theory of health alliances, a budget cap that most Americans rejected, and a tired employer-based and Medicare system. Chapters 10 and 11 will attempt to develop further the constraints and necessities of competition and regulation in health care.

Competition and the Allocation of Resources

How might competition in health care affect the allocation of health care resources? There are several answers to this question, in part, because of disagreement about what constitutes competition in health care. Uwe E. Reinhardt ["Economists in Health Care: Saviors or Elephants in a Porcelain Shop?" *American Economic Review*, 79 (1989): 337–342], for example, once defined competition in terms of price competition among providers, suggesting that competition cannot exist if public and private insurance pays for three-quarters of health care bills. Kenneth J. Arrow ["The Economics of Moral Hazard: Further Comment," *American Economic Review*, 53 (1968): 537–539], like Enthoven, focuses on competition in the insurance industry. Arrow suggests, for example, that insurance need not completely distort the allocation of health care services. Insurers who were actively cost-conscious, for example, rather than passive payers of health care, could improve the allocation of resources.

It appears that, with the increase in the number of managed care plans (described in Chapter 4), some resources have been saved by more vigilant insurer behavior. Chapters 10 and 11 will show, however, that even vigilant insurer behavior does not guarantee optimal allocation of resources in the health care sector.

Competition may improve the allocation of resources and provide for a more efficient system, but it is not clear that competition reduces the rate of increase in health care costs. Competition also does little to reduce inequities in the provision of health care services or reduce the number of uninsured. Competition improves access when it reduces health care insurance premiums. Competition can reduce the rate of return of existing health plans. It can improve quality; it provides for greater consumer choice of health care plans and services; it forces firms to be more innovative in cost containment.

Regulation and the Allocation of Resources

Regulation of price and supply in the health care industry, as in other industries, may create inefficiencies and increase prices. It may also be ineffective insofar as regulated in-patient hospital costs, for example, shift to unregulated out-patient settings. Rather than benefiting the public interest, regulation may benefit the firms or providers that are regulated. If society is concerned about the degree of equity in acquiring health care services, however, a role for government assistance exists.

Health Care Marketplace

The competitive managed care revolution in the 1990s may lead one to forget how acceptable it once was for the state to regulate hospital rates. It was believed that insuring organizations were not considered purchasers of hospital care since they were incapable of controlling costs. The following decision confirms the dominant role of the Health Services Cost Review Commission in controlling hospital costs in the state of Maryland.

Chapter 9 Appendix

277 Md. 93
Blue Cross of Maryland, Inc., et al.,
v.
Franklin Square Hospital et al.

No. 53
Court of Appeals of Maryland.
Decided March 2, 1976

Hospitals filed bill for declaratory judgment challenging portions of regulations governing hospital rate applications promulgated by the Health Services Cost Review Commission (p. 798).

The Act [which established the Maryland Health Services Cost Review Commission] vested the Commission with jurisdiction over the costs and rates of hospitals, health care institutions and related institutions located in Maryland. The Commission was charged with the responsibility of assuring that hospital "rates are set equitably among all purchasers or classes of purchasers without undue discrimination or preference." In order to accomplish this, the Commission was given "full power to review and approve the reasonableness of rates established or requested" by hospitals subject to its jurisdiction. At issue here is the meaning of the terms "purchaser" and "classes of purchasers" as used in the statute. Also at issue is the scope of the Commission's authority to "review and approve" the reasonableness of established or proposed hospital rate structures (pp. 800–801).

The Commission is further to determine that, in each hospital, rates are set equitably among all purchasers or classes of purchasers of services without undue discrimination or preference. Medicare, Blue Cross, Medicaid and private insurance companies are not to be treated by the Commission as purchasers or classes of purchasers within the meaning of the Act. Further, the term "equitably" as used in the Act means fairly—not equally—and the term "all," as used in the Act, means all purchasers or classes of purchasers regardless of the area of the hospital from which they purchase services or the types of services purchased. The term "undue" as used in the Act means not appropriate or suitable, improper, unjustifiable; going beyond what is appropriate, warranted, or natural; excessive (p. 803).

In the event the Commission finds that the rate structure charged or proposed by the hospital is reasonable it shall approve the rates even though some other rate structure might also be reasonable (p. 803).

In sum, we hold that Blue Cross is not a "purchaser" (p. 807).

In our view, the Legislature, in delegating to review and approve the reasonableness of hospital rates, intended that the Commission have the power to approve those rates which it considers best designed to effectuate the purposes of the statute. The Commission is not required, as the hospitals contend, to defer to the hospital's view of reasonableness in cases of conflict. If, in the Commission's opinion, a proposed rate structure is designed to further the purposes of the statute less effectively than another structure would, then it would be proper for the Commission to reject the proposed rates.

The provisions of the Act reflect the legislative intent that the Commission have broad authority over the financial affairs of hospitals and that it should only approve those rates *best* designed to assure fair costs and fiscal integrity (p. 809).

As can be seen, the statute requires the Commission to assure not only that rates are reasonable in light of services and costs, but also that rates be set equitably and without undue discrimination. Under subsection (b) the Commission is granted "full power" to review and approve rate schedules, including the power to disapprove rate schedules, which are already in operation (p. 809).

In light of the provisions of the statute, we agree with the Commission that it is empowered to approve that rate structure which it finds to be most reasonable under the circumstances (p. 810).

10
Technology and Rationing in Health Care

According to most economists, the adoption of new technology has accounted for the largest increase in health care costs between the post-World War II period and the early 1990s [Joseph P. Newhouse, "Medical Care Costs: How Much Welfare Loss?" *Journal of Economic Perspectives*, Summer 1992, pp. 3–21]. At the same time, technology has provided new sight and hearing capabilities, enhanced physical mobility, and has added to the possibilities to extend and improve the quality of life. The increase in the costs of technology may mean considering ways to implicitly and explicitly ration health care services, some of which were introduced by new technology. This chapter, therefore, combines health care technology with the essential economics of health care rationing.

Technology and Rising Health Care Costs

Economists have found it difficult to identify precisely how much of the increase in health care costs is due to increases in technology because, in large part, of the interrelationship between insurance and technology. The introduction of expensive technology raises costs, which engenders increased insurance reimbursement, which may lead to newer technology. Other variables, such as changes in real income and population, may also add to health care costs, but these variables are highly correlated with new technology [J. H. Goddeeris, "Medical Insurance, Technological Change, and Welfare," *Economic Inquiry*, 22 (1984): 56–57; J. H. Goddeeris and B. Weisbord, "What We Don't Know about Why Health Expenditures Have Soared: Interaction of Insurance and Technology," *Mount Sinai Journal of Medicine*, 52 (1985): 685–691]. Researchers have suggested that as much as 50 percent of the increase in hospital costs stems from new technology [R. W. Evans, "Health Care Technology and the Inevitability of Resource Allocation and Rationing Decisions," *Journal of the American Medical Association*, 249 (1983): 2047–2057; W. B. Schwartz, "The Inevitable Failure of Cost Containment Strategies," *Journal of the American Medical*

Association, 257 (1987): pp. 220–224; B. J. Hillman, "Government Health Policy and the Diffusion of New Medical Devices," *Health Services Research*, 21 (1986): 681–711]. Not all new technology leads to rising health care costs, however. For example, the prices of soft contact lenses fell 50 percent between 1971 and 1982 [U.S. Congress, Office of Technology Assessment, *Federal Policies and the Medical Device Industry*, OTA-H-230 (Washington, DC: U.S. Government Printing Office, 1984), pp. 29–30]. Soft contact lenses, however, unlike most other health care technologies, are rarely paid for by insurers.

The implementation of technology affects the average cost curve of the providers of health care. Technology that is cost saving lowers the average cost curve of providers. Technology that improves the process of treatment and some product innovation lowers costs. Technology that is cost increasing, such as some new product discoveries, raises the average cost curve of the provider. In his analysis of rising health care costs, Newhouse [1992] attempted to ascertain the proportion of rising health care costs due to new technology. After systematically examining factors that may have led to increasing health care costs over time—such as increases in the age of the population, increases in real income, and increases in insurance coverage—Newhouse concluded that 50 percent or more of the health care expenditure increase is due to changes in technology. Technology, however, is not endogenous, and it stems, according to Burton A. Weisbrod ["The Health Care Quadrilemma: An Essay on Technological Change, Insurance, Quality of Care, and Cost Containment," *Journal of Economic Literature*, 29 (1991): 523–552] from increased health insurance coverage. Full coverage of kidney dialysis has led to improved kidney dialysis equipment. Coverage of in vitro fertilization has led to new technology in infertility treatments [p. 530]. As technology has increased, expanded insurance coverage has been demanded by patients in order to pay for it. Uncertainty about the benefits and costs of technology increase its use at even a greater rate if patient, physician, and managed care plan are risk adverse. As Mark McClennan suggests ["Uncertainty, Health-Care Technologies, and Health-Care Choices," *American Economic Review*, May 1995, pp. 38–44], a technology that causes mortality in one-third of the cases, in another third has no effect on patients, and in another third has preventive effects is, on average, not beneficial. However, for a subset of patients, the use of the technology may be appropriate. Since insurance and technology are interdependent, a passive or cost-conscious managed care firm has a major effect on the amount and type of technology that is developed. Under the passive insurer, adoption of the latest technology, regardless of costs, is encouraged. Under the cost-conscious insurer, it is discouraged unless long-run costs can be reduced. Weisbrod does not address, however, the incentives of both passive and managed care plans to curtail use of technology in order not to attract high-risk individuals. If high-risk individuals are aware of the superior technology offered at particular hospitals, for example, managed care firms that use these hospitals may begin to suffer financial losses on high-risk enrollees. These incentives may reduce a hospital's demand for the latest technology.

In addition to the relationship of the presence of insurance and the adoption of new technology, new technology also appears to be a function of biomedical research, especially the scientific research conducted by the National Institutes of Health (NIH). David M. Cutler, for example, cites the increases in costs in the treatment of heart attacks which are due to new technology ["Technology, Health Costs, and the NIH," paper prepared for the National Institutes of Health Roundtable on Biomedical Research," September 1995, p. 12]. Most of the basic research for this new technology stems from NIH-funded research.

Diffusion of Medical Technology

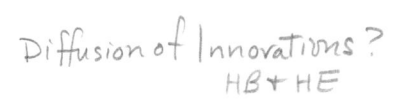

New technology is not immediately adopted by each hospital or health care supplier in an industry. Firms have different capital requirements, purchasing cycles, production functions, and profit levels. Because of reimbursement trends, technology adoption may shift between out-patient and in-patient settings or to a subacute setting outside the hospital environment. L. B. Russell [*Technology in Hospitals: Medical Advances and Their Diffusion* (Washington, DC: Brookings Institution, 1979), pp. 158–159] found that, among hospitals, the more prestigious technologies were more likely to be adopted by the largest hospitals (in terms of number of beds) than by the smallest hospitals.

A. L. Hillman and J. S. Schwartz ["The Adoption and Diffusion of CT and MRI in the United States: A Comparative Analysis," *Medical Care*, 23 (1985): 1283–1294] looked at the adoption and diffusion of computerized axial topography (CT) and magnetic resonance imaging (MRI) devices. They found that in hospital settings, the CT, a diagnostic imaging device, had a much more rapid diffusion rate than the more costly MRI, also a diagnostic imaging device but with no radiation exposure and little patient discomfort. In nonhospital settings, the adoption rate was about the same. Apparently, the uncertainty about whether DRGs would continue to reimburse the capital costs of new equipment delayed a more widespread adoption of the MRI in hospitals. Moreover, more than four years after the introduction of the MRI, only fourteen of seventy Blue Cross plans reimbursed MRI procedures [E. P. Steinberg, J. E. Sisk, and K. E. Locke, "X-Ray CT and Magnetic Resonance Imagers," *New England Journal of Medicine*, 313 (1985): 859–864]. Hillman and Schwartz also reported that most of the hospitals that did purchase MRI units were academic hospitals, which may put greater emphasis on new technology. In addition, Steinberg, Sisk, and Locke suggested that the relatively slow diffusion of the MRI systems might stem from the belief that the incremental marginal benefits for magnetic resonance imagers are relatively less than for CT scanners. Moreover, they report, perhaps due to the DRG reimbursement being limited to in-patient settings, a proportionately greater number of MRIs than CT scanners have been installed in out-patient rather than in-patient areas.

F. A. Sloan, J. Valvona, and J. M. Perrin ["Diffusion of Surgical Technology: An Exploratory Study," *Journal of Health Economics*, 5 (1986): 31–61], in an analysis of five surgical procedures at 521 hospitals between 1971 and 1981, found evidence (although weak) that technology diffusion is more likely to occur in teaching hospitals than in nonteaching hospitals, a conclusion that supports Hillman and Schwartz's findings. According to Sloan, Valvona, and Perrin, payment mechanisms, such as rate setting by states, have had little effect on the pattern of diffusion except for a small negative effect on the use of coronary bypass surgery. Medical technologies may also be used to treat a variety of existing conditions. The laser, for example, was originally developed to be used for ophthalmologic and dermatologic purposes but has also been used for oncology and thoracic surgery patients [Annetine Gelijns and Nathan Rosenberg, "The Dynamics of Technological Change in Medicine," *Health Affairs*, 13 (1994): 28–46, p. 32].

Medicare Reimbursement and Technology

After the implementation of the prospective payment system under DRGs, the federal government treated new capital technology as a pass-through, fully reimbursing each hospital's actual capital expenditures. Since fiscal year 1992, however, the government has been phasing in a prospectively determined rate for hospital capital costs similar to traditional reimbursement of operating costs under the DRG system. By fiscal year 2002, the government will be paying capital costs fully and prospectively, as it currently pays for operating costs. During the phase-in period, hospital-specific costs will be merged with one government capital payment rate [Prospective Payment Assessment Commission, *Medicare and the American Health Care System*, Report to the Congress, June 1996, p. 65]. Total capital costs paid for by Medicare for fiscal year 1996 were approximately $8.8 billion [p. 65]. Similar to payment for operating costs under the DRG system, payments for capital costs will be updated annually. Depending on the stringency of the prospectively based capital DRG, technology adoption might be reduced compared to the time when capital costs were paid on a simple pass-through basis.

The DRG payment system had an effect on the types of technology adopted even before the inclusion of capital costs in the DRG. Since 1982, there have been incentives to adopt technology that would reduce operating costs. There have also been countervailing incentives to adopt technology in order to attract physicians and hospital admissions to the hospital. The adoption by many hospitals of a substantial amount of technology might have led to a higher DRG (even for operating costs) in the periodic governmental review of the DRG weights [Gail R. Wilensky, "Technology as a Culprit and Benefactor," *Quarterly Review of Economics and Business*, 30 (Winter 1990): 45–53].

The Pharmaceutical Industry

Pharmaceutical expenditures in 1995 were approximately $83 billion, or less than 10 percent of all health care expenditures for that year [Katharine R. Levit et al., "National Health Expenditures, 1994," *Health Care Financing Review*, 18 (1996): 175–214, Table 5, p. 185]. (Data reported under "national health expenditures" include "drugs and other medical nondurables"). There were 585 firms in the pharmaceutical industry in 1992, although the drug industry consists of a large number of relevant product markets [U.S. Department of Commerce, Bureau of the Census, *1992 Census of Manufacturers*, Industry Series, p. Drugs 28C-7, Table 1a, June 1995]. Many firms making one type of drug could make other types of pharmaceuticals (the cross-elasticity of supply is high), but patents (which provide a seventeen-year monopoly) mitigate against it and make it difficult for new firms to enter the market.

Pharmaceuticals are not as well covered by insurance as other health care expenses. In 1994, 38 percent of pharmaceutical expenditures, compared to nearly 70 percent of health care expenditures as a whole, were paid by third-party insuring organizations [U.S. Department of Commerce, *Statistical Abstract of the United States, 1996*, Table 162, p. 115]. Many Medicare beneficiaries enrolled in HMOs are now covered for out-patient pharmaceuticals, since approximately 60 percent of Medicare HMOs offer prescription drug benefits (under the traditional Medicare program only in-patient pharmaceuticals are covered) [Carlos Zarabozo et al., "Medicare Managed Care: Numbers and Trends," *Health Care Financing Review*, 17 (1996): 243–255].

Patents, which can retard entry into markets, can also enhance the potential profit stream of firms that have them and in this way encourage research and development. In order to stimulate entry, competition, research and development, the Drug Price Competition and Patent Term Restoration Act was passed in 1984. The Act extended the life of the patent, which is lost during the Food and Drug Administration (FDA) drug review and approval process. In addition, the Act made it easier for generic drug products to enter the market after the expiration of the patent [Henry G. Grabowski and John M. Vernon, "Brand Loyalty, Entry, and Price Competition in Pharmaceuticals After the 1984 Drug Act," *Journal of Law and Economics*, 35 (1992): 331–350].

Some pharmaceuticals have the potential to reduce health care costs. Vaccines for tetanus and poliomyelitis, for example, have been shown to be cost-effective [B. A. Weisbrod and J. Huston, "*Benefits and Costs of Human Vaccines in Developed Countries: An Evaluative Survey*," Report 2 (Washington, DC: Pharmaceutical Manufacturers Association, 1983)]. Likewise, prophylactic antibiotics have been shown to be cost-effective [A. Kaiser, "Antimicrobial Prophylaxis in Surgery," *New England Journal of Medicine*, 315 (1986): 1378–1383]. In contrast, it is not clear that medications are cost-effective in treating hypertension [M. C. Weinstein and W. B. Stason, "Cost-effectiveness of Interventions to Prevent or Treat Coronary Heart Disease," *Annual Review of Public Health*, 6 (1985): 41–63]. Sumatriptan, a pharmaceutical targeted for severe migraine headaches, was found to be cost-effective in a survey of patients who had taken the drug in 1994. Drug expenditures per month increased, but total health care expenditures declined 41 percent after Sumatriptan was begun [Randall F. Legg et al., "Cost-Effectiveness of Sumatriptan in a Managed Care Population," *American Journal of Managed Care*, 3 (1997): 117–122]. In their 1993 review of the published literature of the cost-effectiveness of pharmaceuticals between 1986 and 1991, Douglas Coyle and Michael Drummond conclude that drug interventions are more cost effective than no intervention and at least as effective as alternative interventions ["Does Expenditure on Pharmaceuticals Give Good Value for Money? Current Evidence and Policy Implications," *Health Policy*, 26 (1993): 55–75]. In their review, however, Coyle and Drummond note the difficulties in defining "quality" outcomes as well as finding comparable clinical indicators of patients.

Trends in Health Care Costs

Most studies have shown that, for any given point in time, health maintenance organizations or prepaid capitated plans have lower costs than indemnity plans in the fee-for-service sector, even after adjusting for the case mix of the enrolled population (see Chapter 4).

Two longitudinal studies (from 1961 to 1974 and from 1976 to 1981), however, showed that the rate of increase in HMO costs is about the same as the rate of increase in fee-for-service costs [H. S. Luft, "Trends in Medical Care Costs," *Medical Care*, 18 (1980): 1–16; J. P. Newhouse, W. B. Schwartz, A. P. Williams, and C. Witsberger, "Are Fee-for-Service Costs Increasing Faster than HMO Costs?" *Medical Care*, 23 (1985): 960–966]. Since health maintenance organizations at a single point in time have lower costs than fee-for-service organizations, similar rates of increase imply slightly greater absolute increases in costs in the fee-for-service sector. Newhouse, Schwartz, Williams and Witsberger suggest that this trend in health care costs may be due to the fee-for-service sector's greater use of technology, but they suggest that HMOs also appear to be adopting most of the new technology. A later study by J. P. Newhouse ["Has the Erosion of the Medical Marketplace Ended?" *Competition in the Health Care Sector: Ten Years Later*, ed. W. Greenberg (Durham, NC: Duke University Press, 1988), pp. 41–56] also shows that much of the increase in health care costs is due to the adoption of new technology. W. B. Schwartz ["The Inevitable Failure of Cost Containment Strategies," *Journal of the American Medical Association*, 257 (1987): 220–224] similarly finds that the adoption and diffusion of new technology is largely responsible for rising health care costs. In contrast, variables such as the aging of the population and the costs of malpractice insurance have had inconsequential effects.

At least two reasons explain why the adoption of new technology continues to increase. First, as this chapter has suggested, even partial regulatory controls of technology under Medicare were not put into place until 1992. Second, and more important, patients demand the implementation of medically efficacious practices and procedures regardless of their economic efficiency [W. B. Schwartz and P. L. Joskow, "Medical Efficacy versus Economic Efficiency," *New England Journal of Medicine*, 299 (1978): 1452–1464].

An example may show the difference between medically efficacious and economically efficient practices and procedures. Suppose physicians were able to determine with certainty the potential marginal benefits and costs of the utilization of new technologies. Assume that the marginal benefits from using a new technology were worth $500, including the increased value of life from successful medical intervention, assuming that a monetary value can be assessed. Assume that the marginal costs were $400, including the pecuniary costs of the procedure, the cost of pain, and the costs of waiting and inconvenience (assuming that the latter costs can be valued). Physicians, in this case, would perform the test or procedure because it would be medically efficacious. Economists, in this case, would agree with the physicians' course of action because marginal benefits would exceed marginal costs and the procedure would be economically efficient. Suppose, however, that the marginal benefits were calculated to be zero with no uncertainty, and the marginal costs of the procedure were determined to be $500. Ethical physicians would not perform the procedure since it would not be medically efficacious and no benefits would accrue to the patient. Economists would agree with the medical decision because marginal costs outweigh any marginal benefits. The procedure would also not be economically efficient.

Medical efficacy and economic efficiency conflict when the marginal costs of a procedure are $500 and the marginal benefits are greater than zero but less than $500. Physicians would normally go ahead with the procedure since there are some positive benefits; the procedure would be considered medically efficacious. Economists, in contrast, would view the procedure as inefficient because marginal costs exceed marginal benefits. According to Schwartz and Joskow, in a large number of procedures marginal costs exceed marginal benefits yet the benefits are greater than zero. Physicians find it difficult to refrain from ordering or performing the procedures because the patient benefits from them, but from society's standpoint they are economically inefficient.

Schwartz similarly finds that the adoption and diffusion of new technology is largely responsible for rising health care costs [William B. Schwartz, "The Inevitable Failure of Cost Containment Strategies," *Journal of the American Medical Association*, 257 (1987): 220–224], and he suggests three reasons. As technology develops it may become less invasive; therefore, using degree of pain as a cost, technology makes undergoing treatment less costly. Second, Schwartz suggests that many new technologies cannot substitute for previous technologies; once a technology has been used, a new, perhaps superior technology does not automatically replace it. Schwartz provides the example of the MRI not replacing the CT entirely, in part because the MRI is not suitable for those who suffer from claustrophobia. Third, Schwartz suggests that even if the costs of the procedure are reduced through economies of scale or reduced through its availability on an out-patient basis, the increase in volume of procedures may increase total costs.

Schwartz and Mendelson point to a number of examples where the expectation of new advances in medicine that would have positive benefits eventually increased costs [William B. Schwartz and Daniel N. Mendelson, "Why Managed Care Cannot Contain Hospital Costs—Without Rationing," *Health Affairs*, Summer 1992, pp. 100–107]. These technologies include the implantable cardiac defibrillator for cardiac arrhythmias, erythropoietin for the treatment of anemia, and different contrast media for safer radiologic studies. Mendelson and Schwartz predict that these technologies alone will add $5 billion annually to health care costs. In a study of high-cost diseases such as breast cancer, heart disease, ulcers and pneumonia over the period 1971–1981 [Anne A. Scitovsky, "Changes in the Costs of Treatment of Selected Illnesses, 1971–1981," *Medical Care*, 23 (1985): 1345–1357], Scitovsky found that the big increases in costs came from expensive new technology rather than the use of ancillary services, which were the major source of cost increases in her previous study periods of 1951–1964 and 1964–1971.

Gelijns and Rosenberg examine the procedures of laparoscopic cholecystectomy that have the possibility of substantially reducing unit costs but nevertheless increased costs because its use included not only sicker but mildly symptomatic and high-risk patients [Gelijns and Rosenberg p. 39]. Therefore, David Cutler notes, the number of individuals receiving laparoscopic cholecystetomy increased by 57 percent between 1988 and 1992, resulting in higher per-person expenditures for gallbladder disease ["Technology, Health Costs, and the NIH," unpublished paper prepared for the National Institutes of Health Economics Roundtable on Biomedical Research, September 1995, p. 16].

Because of the conflict between medical efficacy and economic efficiency, phrases such as unnecessary surgery and unnecessary hospitalization are vague and ambiguous. The economist considers surgery or hospitalization that does not pass a cost-benefit test unnecessary. The physician and the insured patient (both of whom are unconcerned about pecuniary cost) do not consider surgery unnecessary unless the benefits are virtually zero. The conflict between medical efficacy and economic efficiency can be seen most vividly in *Wickline v. California* [192 Cal. App. 3d 1630, 236 Cal. Rptr. 810, (1986)]. In that case, a Medicaid patient, Lois Wickline, was admitted to a hospital in California for surgery for circulatory and vascular ailments. After she developed problems from the surgery, her physician requested Medicaid approval for an additional eight days in the hospital. Medi-Cal, the California state Medicaid agency, would approve an additional stay of only four days. After Wickline's discharge, she developed increased circulatory problems that culminated in the surgical removal of her leg. Wickline sued the Medi-Cal authorities for refusing to pay for the length of stay recommended by her doctor.

The California Second District Court of Appeals ruled that, in fact, the Medi-Cal officials had good and valid medical reasons to believe that the additional four days were unnecessary, and they were exonerated from any legal responsibility in this case. The most important part of the decision, however, was that third-party payers could be held responsible for refusing to pay for hospital stays and medical procedures in which there are some potential benefits to be gained. That is, as long as there are benefits for the individual, third parties cannot refuse to pay for procedures, even though society might value these benefits at less than the marginal costs. If procedures in which costs exceed nonzero benefits make up an increasing portion of health care expenditures, public policy may have to consider explicit rationing as a supplement to competition and regulation, to contain rising health care costs.

The Wickline case illustrates two important issues in health care. The first is that the legal system can help improve the quality of care in insuring organizations. That is, insuring organizations, understanding the possibility of a legal suit that can make them potentially liable for millions of dollars in addition to potential unfavorable publicity, have strong incentives to be cautious before refusing to pay for treatment that has positive benefits. Implementation of the law provides that a certain level of quality will be maintained. The law, however, is an imperfect instrument to ensure quality for a number of reasons. First, legal actions can be expensive to undertake, although some lawyers are willing to work on a contingency fee basis. Second, individuals may not know when to initiate suits, especially under the stress of health concerns. Third, under the Employee Retirement Income Security Act of 1974, it is not clear that the 44 million individuals enrolled in insuring organizations that are offered by self-funded employers (ERISA plans) will fall under the provisions of the *Wickline* decision. [Mary Ann Chirba-Martin and Troyen A. Brennan, "The Critical Role of ERISA in State Health Reform," *Health Affairs*, 13 (1994): 142–156, p. 151]. See also William P. Peters and Mark C. Rogers, "Variation in Approval by Insurance Companies of Coverage for Autologous Bone Marrow Transplantation for Breast Cancer," *New England Journal of Medicine*, 330 (1994): 473–477, and Wendy K. Mariner, "State Regulation of Managed Care and the Employee Retirement Income Security Act," *New England Journal of Medicine*, 335 (1996): 1986–1990]. Recently, however, Texas passed the first state law that allows patients to sue a managed care plan for malpractice. It is unclear, however, that this law can be applied to ERISA plans ["Texas Will Allow Malpractice Suits Against HMOs," *New York Times*, June 5, 1997, pp. A1, A22].

Rationing

Because of unlimited demand for limited resources, goods, and services, rationing, or the process of the allocation of resources, takes place in every area of the economy, including health care. The price system is the usual method of rationing goods and services. In competitive industries, price equals the marginal cost of providing goods and services. The price system has the advantage of being completely impersonal and requiring no government intervention. For example, the price of a VCR at a particular store may be $150. Individuals can purchase a VCR at this price regardless of their race, gender, or age, the time they spent waiting in line, or their degree of influence or bargaining power with the store owner. Only those without $150 cannot purchase the VCR. The same concept applies to most other goods and services. Society does not appear to be too concerned if some individuals cannot afford a VCR. For services like health care, on the other hand, society is concerned that all individuals receive at least some basic level of services.

Nonprice Rationing in Other Industries

Although the price system is the most efficient way of allocating goods and services, it is not always used in other industries. For example, although Super Bowl tickets have a face value price of perhaps $200, a football fan may pay more than ten times that amount. In addition, a buyer may need friends and contacts to be able to obtain the tickets even at that higher price. Super Bowl tickets may, therefore, be allocated on a price basis (but at a much higher price than the face price of a ticket) as well as by the contacts of individual buyers.

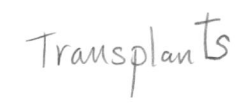

Rent control has been in force in some form for a large number of apartments in New York City since 1943. Apparently, rents are held below the equilibrium level; long waiting lists are established for the rent-controlled apartments. Thus, the rationing of apartments in New York is based on the rent that is charged and on the inclination of individuals to endure a substantial delay before obtaining an apartment as well as on contacts who may know of an apartment's availability.

Many goods and services may be rationed on a geographic basis in addition to a price basis. It is more costly, for example, in terms of time (opportunity cost) and transportation costs for an individual in, say, Philadelphia to see a Broadway show than for someone who lives in New York City. Rationing of incoming freshman slots at universities may be based on high school academic performance and standardized test scores in addition to being able to pay tuition. Rationing of the "best tables" in a restaurant may be based on the repeat business and stature of customers in addition to the size of the tip to the maitre d'.

Nonprice Rationing in Health Care

With success in the outcomes of solid organ transplantation, it is not surprising to find an increasing number of individuals who have been put on the list as possible recipients of organs such as liver, heart, and lungs. The United Network for Organ Sharing (UNOS), a private nonprofit firm responsible to the government, found, at the end of October 1996, nearly 50,000 patient registrants for solid organs [Paul J. Hauptman and Kevin J. O'Connor, "Procurement and Allocation of Solid Organs for Transplantation," *New England Journal of Medicine*, 336 (1997): 422–431, p. 422]. All potential recipients of donated organs are put on the UNOS directory. Potential kidney recipients, for example, are allocated cadaveric kidneys based on the following criteria: (1) patients must be on a local waiting list; (2) time on the waiting list; (3) quality of match; (4) medical urgency; (5) "logistical score", or ease and rapidity of performance of the transplant [James F. Childress, "Ethical Criteria for Procuring and Distributing Organs for Transplantation," in *Organ Transplantation Policy Issues and Prospects*, ed. James F. Blumstein and Frank A. Sloan (Chapel Hill, NC: Duke University Press, 1989) p. 104]. Liver and heart transplants are based mostly on medical urgency and waiting time, while lung, heart-lung, and pancreatic transplants emphasize waiting time [Hauptman and O'Connor, p. 427].

As Blumstein and Sloan suggest, the allocation of human organs is the primary exception to the emphasis on a competitive price system in health care. Ethical, equity, and distributional objectives apparently supersede price in allocating the purchase and sale of human organs. In addition, demand for human organs far exceeds the supply which, if unchecked, would drive up the price to an extremely high level. Indeed, the commercial sale of organs is prohibited by law. In 1995, however, there were 19,136 kidney-pancreas, kidney, pancreas, liver, heart, heart-lung, and lung transplants, while 47,970 registrants were listed as of August 1996 [United Network for Organ Sharing, "U.S. Waiting List Statistics," http://www.traders.co.UK/insulintrust/unos.htm, pp. 1, 2].

Nonprice rationing is not uncommon in the health care sector. Not everyone in the United States receives "presidential medicine." As V. R. Fuchs points out ["The Rationing of Medical Care," *New England Journal of Medicine*, 311 (1984): 1572–1573], health care may be rationed on a geographic basis because physicians are much more scarce (and traveling time to see a physician is therefore greater) in Montana, for example, than in New York. The care in quality hospitals may also be rationed by nonprice mechanisms. Although hospitals are generally covered by insurance, not all surgery goes on at university hospitals that many perceive to be of superior quality or at "brand name" hospitals such as the Cleveland Clinic or the Mayo Clinic.

Within a specific disease, there has been explicit rationing in the United States. Kidney disease, for example, may be treated by traditional dialysis, continuous ambulatory peritoneal dialysis, or transplantation, depending in large part on the physical condition of the patient. According to P. J. Held ["Access to Kidney Transplantation," *Archives of Internal Medicine*, 148 (1988): 2594–2600], among those recommended for kidney transplantation there appears to be explicit rationing based on race, gender, age, health condition, and income. Patients who are white, male, young, nondiabetic, and high income have a greater likelihood of receiving a kidney transplant than other patients. Held speculates that perhaps blacks prefer dialysis over transplantation because, in fact, blacks do better than whites on regular dialysis. The willingness of relatives to donate kidneys may also be greater among whites than among blacks. In addition, although Medicare pays for the entire cost of transplantation, Medicare did not pay for outpatient drugs during the time frame of the Held study (1980 to 1985) and still does not pay for transportation to and from the transplantation hospital. This, of course, means that low-income people are less likely to choose transplants.

The rationing of a limited number of suitable kidneys may also reflect a bias of white male physicians who identify with white patients or who believe that black patients may be at greater risk in kidney transplants because of their more common ailments of hypertension and diabetes. The University of Pittsburgh has been less haphazard in allocating the cadaver kidneys in its hospital. The hospital has assigned points based on waiting time, antigen matching, antibody analysis, medical urgency, and logistical practicality. Each potential patient receives points based on these criteria. [T. E. Starzl et al., "X-Ray CT and Magnetic Resonance Imagers," *New England Journal of Medicine*, 313 (1987): 859–864].

Medicare's decision to pay for kidney dialysis enabled a greater number of people to utilize this service, thereby reducing the financial and emotional burden on family members. The result has been a large increase in the costs of treating kidney disease victims. In 1974, the first year that Medicare was responsible for end-stage renal disease (ESRD) victims, expenditures were $229 million for 16,000 individuals [Paul W. Eggers, "Trends in Medicare Reimbursement for End-Stage Renal Disease: 1974–1979," *Health Care Financing Review*, 6 (1984): 31–38, p. 33]. By 1994, there were 242,000 Medicare beneficiaries with ESRD at a cost of $8.2 billion ["High-Cost Users of Medicare Services," *Health Care Financing Review*, Medicare and Medicaid Statistical Supplement, 1996, p. 32].

In 1988, more than 900 individuals awaited a heart transplant in the United States. Most individuals who received transplants were males more than 45 years old. Eighty-four percent of all recipients were white (U.S. General Accounting Office, *Heart Transplants, Concerns about Cost, Access, and Availability of Donor Organs* (Washington, DC: U.S. Government Printing Office, 1989)]. It is not clear why this is so. Perhaps white patients, who in general have higher incomes than nonwhites and are more apt to be insured, more easily meet the hospital's financial criteria. Perhaps also because whites live longer than nonwhites, they are more apt to develop heart disease that eventually dictates heart transplantation. According to the U.S. General Accounting Office study, hospitals used both medical and financial criteria in selecting transplant patients. The survey of eighteen hospitals found that individuals who had end-stage heart disease and who could not benefit from any other medical or surgical procedures were the first to be selected. In regard to financial criteria, three of the eighteen hospitals reported that transplant surgery could not begin unless payment was assured. Fourteen hospitals said that some patients would be accepted without payment. One hospital did not provide its views on financial criteria.

The state of Oregon is the first public entity in the United States to attempt explicit rationing of procedures for its Medicaid patients. To extend basic Medicaid coverage to 1,500 additional individuals, the state eliminated coverage of bone marrow, heart, liver, and pancreas transplantation. These transplants were projected to cost approximately $2.2 million for 34 patients between 1987 and 1989 [H. G. Welch and E. B. Larson, "The Oregon Decision to Curtail Funding for Organ Transplantation," *New England Journal of Medicine*, 319 (1988): 171–173; "Rising Cost of Medical Treatment Forces Oregon to 'Play God'," *Washington Post*, February 5, 1988, p. A-1]. Apparently eliminating only the most expensive transplant procedures from coverage, Oregon still covers the less expensive procedures, such as cornea and kidney transplants, under the state Medicaid provisions. In addition, individuals can still use commercial insurance to pay for coverage, can solicit donations, or can move to another state in order to receive a rationed transplant.

An even more ambitious rationing scheme by the state of Oregon is its ranking of 1,600 medical procedures by priority of treatment. In this ranking system, the costs of the procedure are weighed against the benefits. The benefits are calculated as the number of years the patient would live longer, multiplied by a "quality of well-being" index. This index, agreed on by a number of health experts, is based on such subjective criteria as the time before the ailment could recur and the patient's health after treatment ["Oregon Lists Illnesses by Priority to See Who Gets Medicaid Care," *New York Times*, May 3, 1990, p. 1]. Some preliminary reports, however, suggest that the rationing program may have had some undesirable effects on health care services delivered. An increase in low-birth-weight infants as well as a reduction in "prenatal care" have been reported. These results may reflect the relative newness of the rationing program as well as more complete data on the health status of the poor ["Oregon Plan Covering Medicaid Patients Is Off to Rough Start," *Modern Healthcare*, September 4, 1995, p. 90].

Rationing health care by age may be another form of nonprice rationing. Researchers have examined health care expenditures for the aged population relative to expenditures for the nonaged population. C. R. Fisher ["Differences by Age Groups in Health Care Spending," *Health Care Financing Review*, 1 (1980) 4: 65–90] found that persons who are older than 65 incur 29 percent of all health care expenditures but represent only 11 percent of the population. Moreover, Fisher found that in 1978 the average annual medical expenses for those age 65 and over were $2,026, compared to $764 for individuals age 19 to 64 and $286 for individuals under age 19. In a later, closely related study, M. L. Berk et al. ["How the U.S. Spends Its Health Care Dollar," *Health Care Financing Review*, 8 (1988) 3: 69–82] found that 1 percent of the population accounted for 29 percent of health care expenditures and that more than 43 percent of this group was over the age of 65. Clearly, reducing care to an elderly population would save a substantial sum of money. Yet rationing by age is also subjective. For example, at what age does rationing begin? Should all procedures be rationed? Should health status along with age be taken into account in the rationing process?

Still another form of nonprice rationing is the termination of life through advanced directives or termination of futile life-prolonging treatment. However, a study by Lawrence J. Schneiderman et al. of the effects of advanced directives on costs showed no effect ["Effects of Offering Advance Directives on Medical Treatments and Costs," *Annals of Internal Medicine*, 117 (1992): 599–606], and a study by Joan M. Teno et al. showed that eliminating "futile" care would have only a modest effect on costs, ["Prognosis-Based Futility Guidelines: Does Anyone Win?" *Journal of the American Geriatrics Society*, 42 (1994): 1202–1207].

Nonprice rationing in health care has always existed in the United States and will continue to exist in the future. The extent and types of rationing in the future will depend on the rate of increase in health care expenditures, the amount and type of new technology, and the demand for the limited supply of body organs.

Health Care Marketplace

The court in *Wickline* found California's Medicaid program (Medi-Cal) responsible for refusing to authorize procedures that could provide potential potential benefits to patients. To the extent that the thrust of the Wickline decision can be applied to other third-party payers, managed care firms will undoubtedly review a person's condition more carefully before denial of treatment is determined.

Chapter 10 Appendix

**192 Cal. App. 3d 1630
Lois J. Wickline, Plaintiff
and Respondent,
v.
State of California, Defendant
and Appellant.**

No. B010156
Court of Appeals, Second District, Division 5
Decided July 30, 1986

Responding to concerns about the escalating cost of health care, public and private payers have in recent years experimented with a variety of cost containment mechanisms. We deal here with one of those programs: The prospective utilization review process (p. 811).

In the cost containment program in issue in this case, prospective utilization review, authority for the rendering of health care services must be obtained before medical care is rendered. Its purpose is to promote the well recognized public interest in controlling health care costs by reducing unnecessary services while still intending to assure that appropriate medical and hospital services are provided to the patient in need. However, such a cost containment strategy creates new and added pressures on the quality assurance portion of the utilization review mechanism. The stakes, the risks at issue, are much higher when a prospective cost containment review process is utilized than when a retrospective review process is used (p. 811).

It is conceded that at all times in issue in this case, the plaintiff was eligible for medical benefits under California's medical assistance program, the "Medi-Cal Act," which is more commonly referred to as Medi-Cal (p. 812).

Wickline was scheduled to be discharged on January 16, 1977. On or about January 16, 1977, Dr. Polonsky concluded that "it was medically necessary" that plaintiff remain in the hospital for an additional eight days beyond her then scheduled discharge date (p. 813).

Dr. Polonsky cited many reasons for his feeling that it was medically necessary for plaintiff to remain in an acute care hospital for an additional eight days, such as the danger of infection and/or clotting (p. 813).

Dr. Glassman rejected Wickline's treating physician's request for an eight-day hospital extension and, instead, authorized an additional four days of hospital stay beyond the originally scheduled discharge date (p. 814).

Dr. Polonsky testified that at the time in issue he felt that Medi-Cal Consultants had the State's interest more in mind than the patient's welfare and that that belief influenced his decision not to request a second extension of Wickline's hospital stay. In addition, he felt that Medi-Cal had the power to tell him, as a treating doctor, when a patient must be discharged from the hospital (p. 815).

Wickline testified that in the first few days after she arrived home she started feeling pain in her right leg and the leg started to lose color (p. 816).

Dr. Polonsky could not estimate when the infection in Wickline's leg first developed after her January 21st discharge from Van Nuys nor did he know when the clotting in that leg first started (p. 816).

In Dr. Polonsky's opinion, to a reasonable medical certainty, had Wickline remained in the hospital for the eight additional days, as originally requested by him and her other treating doctors, she would not have suffered the loss of her leg (p. 817).

Dr. Polonsky testified that in his medical opinion, the Medi-Cal Consultant's rejection of the requested eight-day extension of acute care hospitalization and his authorization of a four-day extension in its place did not conform to the usual medical standards as they existed in 1977 (p. 817).

The patient who requires treatment and who is harmed when care which should have been provided is not provided should recover for the injuries suffered from all those responsible for the deprivation of such care, including, when appropriate, health care payers. Third party payors of health care services can be held legally accountable when medically inappropriate decisions result from defects in the design or implementation of cost containment mechanisms as, for example, when appeals made on a patient's behalf for medical or hospital care are arbitrarily ignored or unreasonably disregarded or overridden. However, the physician who complies without protest with the limitations imposed by a third-party payer, when his medical judgment dictates otherwise, cannot avoid his ultimate responsibility for his patient's care. He cannot point to the health care payer as the liability scapegoat when the consequences of his own determinative medical decisions go sour (p. 819).

The California Legislature's intent, in enacting the Medi-Cal Act, was to provide "mainstream" medical care to the indigent (p. 820).

While we recognize, realistically, that cost consciousness has become a permanent feature of the health care system, it is essential that cost limitation programs not be permitted to corrupt medical judgment. We have concluded, from the facts in issue here, that in this case it did not (p. 820).

11
Insights from Canada, Israel, and the Netherlands

Canada, Israel, and the Netherlands each use different degrees of market competition, government intervention, and rationing in the health care marketplace. Canada differs most from the United States in its reliance on a single-payer rather than a multipayer system. Both Israel and the Netherlands have a multipayer system but put greater stress on distributional equity than does the United States. None of the three countries makes use of the employer in the provision of health insurance. An analysis of each of the three systems will explain the relative doses of competition, regulation, and rationing that might be used in the financing of health care in the United States.

In Canada, the government in each of the ten provinces is a monopoly financing mechanism and a monopsonist buyer of health care services. There is limited nonprice competition among physicians and among hospitals. Unlike the United States, there is greater stress on distributional equity in the health care system and less stress on efficiency.

Israel, a small country with a population of 5.5 million people and an early socialist regulatory tradition, has moved increasingly toward managed competition within a highly regulated framework. The system was formalized with the enactment of the Israeli National Health Insurance Law of 1995. Distributional equity is a major concern, but efficiency is increasingly stressed.

Similar to Israel, the Netherlands has a history of regulation in health care. It has also moved toward a sophisticated system of managed competition in the acute care sector with heavy stress on distributional equity. An understanding of the Dutch health care system illustrates the tensions between achieving distributional equity and efficiency in health care systems today.

Canadian Health Care System

The most important aspect of the Canadian health care system is its single-payor financing system. With a single-payer system, the ten Canadian provinces determine the level of reimbursement, what will be covered under reimbursement, and the amount of cost containment. Consumer choice is removed from the set of determinants of cost containment in the marketplace. The single-payer system, however, has an important advantage over a multipayor system. In Canada, the government runs the single-payer system and has a commitment to universal health care coverage. Thus, there is no evidence of discrimination against high-risk individuals. It is still possible, with budget constraints, for the government to discriminate against high-risk individuals, but the incentives appear to be far weaker when there is no competition among health plans.

The Canadian health care system has no copayments or deductibles to limit care, and the benefit package is substantial, including mental health benefits, pharmaceuticals, and dental care for children under the age of 18. There are no private sector alternatives in Canada, so individuals cannot have a different kind of benefit package or insuring organization, although in some provinces individuals can make out-of-pocket payments to some physicians and hospitals [John K. Iglehart, "Canada's Health Care System Faces Its Problems," *New England Journal of Medicine*, 322 (1990): 562–568]. Health care expenditures in Canada are financed by general taxes.

Although payment for health care services is financed by the government, the suppliers of health care services, including physicians and hospitals, practice and deliver health care services privately (although hospitals must be not-for-profit). Physicians may compete among themselves based on perceived quality or degree of access or any other dimension, but the prices they charge are set by the government. Hospitals also compete on a nonprice quality or access basis. Patients may choose any physician or hospital they desire.

Physicians are generally paid on a fee-for-service basis, but provinces have begun to bundle many fees into a single office visit. In general, if physician costs are greater than a budgeted amount in a period, physician fees are reduced in the subsequent period. Hospitals receive a budget for capital and a budget for operating costs. However, there are almost no government controls on utilization inside or outside the hospital [Robert G. Evans et al., "Controlling Health Expenditures—The Canadian Reality," *New England Journal of Medicine*, 320 (1989): 571–577].

Canada regulates closely the supply of health care facilities. Canada limits the number of hospitals and hospital beds and the number of physicians. Unlike the philosophy of competition based on market forces, the policy of the Canadian government is that a greater supply will generate a greater demand and therefore a greater utilization of health care services.

Health care costs, however, are growing in Canada at a rate greater than most other industrialized countries. In 1994, Canada spent 9.8 percent of its GDP on health care, an increase from 7.4 percent in 1980 and 9.5 percent in 1990, or a greater percentage of its GDP than any other country except the United States [U.S. Department of Commerce, *Statistical Abstract of the United States, 1996*, October 1996, Table 1332, p. 834]. Canada, like every other advanced society, must contend with the cost of new technologies and a growing elderly population.

There is also nonprice rationing of health care in Canada, including long waits for simple coronary bypass heart operations as well as for organ transplants, long waits to be admitted to the hospital, and the compromises on quality of care that such constraints engender. In contrast, lengths of stay at Canadian hospitals are much longer than those in U.S. hospitals. The hospital administrator with a global budget wants to keep individuals in the hospital for a longer period of time because the later days of a hospital visit are usually less costly. Canada also has more hospital admissions than does the United States [Donald A. Redelmeier and Victor R. Fuchs, "Hospital Expenditures in the United States and Canada," *New England Journal of Medicine*, 328 (1993): 772–778]. This creates very high occupancy rates in hospitals, which in turn may create long waiting lines for admission. Since there is no private insurance for high-income individuals, some patients elect to go to medical centers in the United States, close to the Canadian border.

It is difficult to measure the quality of care Canadians receive from their health care system. The 1990 life expectancy of Canadian males of 73.8 years and females of 80.4 years, however, is greater by almost two years than the life expectancy of American males and females. Infant mortality of 6.8 per 1,000 live births is substantially lower than the 9.1 infant mortality rate in the United States [Tom Rathwell, "Health Care in Canada: A System in Turmoil," *Health Policy*, 24 (1994): 5–17]. Of course, genetic and environmental reasons may explain the greater longevity and lower infant mortality statistics in Canada.

It has been suggested that the administrative costs of the Canadian health care system are much lower than the costs of the U.S. system [David U. Himmelstein and S. Woolhandler, "Cost Without Benefit: Administrative Waste in U.S. Health Care," *New England Journal of Medicine*, 314 (1986): 441–445; Redelmeimer and Fuchs (1993)]. But administrative costs may include the costs of additional resources for utilization review and general cost containment in which all managed care firms engage. Without these administrative costs, expenditures for health care would be much higher. Moreover, beyond utilization review, higher administrative costs are associated with a competitive system in which one may choose among many payors and providers of health care services.

Israeli Health Care System

Although, as in Canada, the current health care system in Israel stresses distributional equity of health care services, it is markedly different in many respects from the Canadian system.

Israeli Health Care System Prior to 1995

Prior to 1995, the Israeli health care system consisted of competition among four managed care plans (or "sick funds", as they are termed in Israel), although one of the four, Kupat Holim Klalit, a staff model health maintenance organization, had a dominant market share of approximately 64 percent, while the other three (each of which are IPA-model organizations), Maccabi, Leumit, and Meuhedet, had approximate market shares of 19 percent, 9 percent, and 9 percent, respectively, at the end of 1994 [Bruce Rosen and Reuven Steiner, "Recent Trends in Sick Fund Market Shares," JDC-Brookdale Institute, Jerusalem, October 1996, p. 2]. Each of the four HMOs serves many geographic regions across the entire country.

The Klalit had the dominant share for two main reasons. The first is that the Klalit was willing to enroll any individual, regardless of health status or age. The three other managed care plans competed in part by seeking only younger individuals in good health; the Klalit, with its socialist-labor tradition, was reluctant to compete on this basis. Second, the Klalit was tied to the Histadrut General Federation of Labor; a person who joined the labor federation was automatically a member of Klalit. The Histadrut consisted of more than 60 percent of the Israeli labor force, including its ownership of manufacturing and service industries [Gabi Bin-Nun and David P. Chinitz, "The Roles of Government and the Market in the Israeli Health Care System in the 1980's," in *The Changing Roles of Government and the Market in Health Care Systems*, ed. David P. Chinitz and Marc A. Cohen, JDC-Brookdale Institute, Ministry of Health, November 1993, p. 128]. Moreover, the three other managed care plans had strong incentives to enroll higher-income individuals because premiums paid to the sick funds were based on income [Rosen and Steiner, p. 3].

Beyond cream-skimming practices, the sick funds competed on geographic convenience. For example, the Klalit had more than 1,300 clinics, and 2,300 primary care physicians and owned more than one-third of all hospital beds throughout the country [Bruce Rosen, *The Netanyahu Commission Report: Background, Contents, and Initial Reactions*, Revised Edition JDC-Brookdale, Institute, Jerusalem, December 1991, p. 1]. Maccabi, especially, competed on service, efficiency, and choice of physician.

The sick funds received approximately 50 percent of their monies from employer contributions, 40 percent from premiums and copayments, and 10 percent from government subsidies to the poor and new immigrants [Bruce

Rosen and Avi Y. Ellencweig, *A Mapping of Health Care Reimbursement in Israel*, JDC-Brookdale Institute, Jerusalem, 1988, p. 56].

Hospitals were reimbursed on a per diem basis on rates established by the Ministry of Health. Physician reimbursement was a function largely of negotiations between the Israel Medical Association and the Ministry of Health, Klalit, and the Hadassah Medical Organization. Hospital-based physicians were paid salaries. The Klalit, which employed the most physicians, paid its physicians primarily on a salary basis with extra payments for seeing more patients. Most of Maccabi's physicians were reimbursed on a fee-for-service basis [Rosen and Ellencweig, pp. 8, 9, 13].

There were concerns that a two-tier method of financing had developed, with most of the younger and middle-income population joining the non-Klalit HMOs. Moreover, the uninsured rate in Israel was 4 percent, with no guarantee of universal coverage. It was not against the law for the sick funds to reject new applicants. Long lines were reported for many hospital services. The Ministry of Health owned approximately 40 percent of all hospital beds and was believed to be inefficient. The dominant role of the Klalit and its tie-in to Histadrut, as well as the continued cream skimming of the other sick funds, reduced efficiency-based competition. Physicians were believed to be underpaid, and frequent strikes disrupted the delivery of health care [Rosen, *The Netanyahu Commission Report*, pp. 3–4]. Health care expenditures as a percent of GDP also climbed from 7.6 percent in 1988–1989 to an estimated 8.4 percent in 1994 [State of Israel, Ministry of Health, *Health in Israel*, Jerusalem, 1996, p. 127].

Israeli Health Care System Reforms

After a number of proposals to reform the Israeli health care system, a state judicial commission of inquiry, the Netanyahu Commission (named after the head of the commission, Chief Judge Shoshanna Netanyahu), issued its report in 1990. The report formed the basis for the Israeli health care reforms and the basis of the current Israeli health care system.

The current system consists of managed competition with universal coverage as its main framework. Funding for the system is derived from a 5 percent tax on employers and employees [communication from Bruce Rosen, JDC-Brookdale Institute, Jerusalem, July 15, 1997]. The four existing HMOs, which by law must be nonprofit, continue to compete against one another, but the Klalit no longer has ties to the Histadrut. Competition, however, does not occur on all dimensions of price and quality. The health maintenance organizations cannot compete on price because the premiums of all health maintenance organizations are set at zero by the Ministry of Health. Although the HMOs can compete by paying physicians more or less, the hospitals are reimbursed directly by the Ministry of Health at a set per diem rate. In 1995, the Government instituted a cap on total hospital spending. Hospital spending could not increase more than 2 percent above the increase in per diem rate [communication from Bruce Rosen]. Fifteen procedures are paid on an American-style DRG basis [Bin-Nun and Chinitz, p. 137]. In addition, the government regulates the number of hospitals that can enter the market as well as the technological equipment hospitals can purchase. Entry of new HMOs is barred unless they can achieve additional governmental funding—no new insuring organization has entered since the founding of the state. The Klalit still owns 30 percent of all hospital beds, to which it may refer Klalit patients, the Ministry of Health owns 47 percent, and the remainder are nonprofit or private [David P. Chinitz, "Reforming the Israeli Health Care Market," *Social Science and Medicine*, 39 (1994): 1447–1457, p. 1450]. Under the health care reforms, all government hospitals are to convert to independent status, but this has not yet taken place.

How do the sick funds compete? Since there is no price competition, the HMOs have attempted to improve their perceived quality, to improve service, to increase advertising, and to increase cream skimming. Benefit packages are uniform, however, which limits cream skimming. The HMOs receive a risk adjustment payment from the government, which also helps deter cream skimming. The risk adjustment measure is currently adjusted only by age; other determinants of hospital and physician use will have to be further developed. Individuals may also purchase supplemental insurance coverage for noncovered, noncore services, although the government closely regulates the supplemental market. There are specific diseases, such as Gaucher's disease, that are not part of the sick fund coverage package but are funded retrospectively by the government.

Most cost containment stems from the government-imposed cap on the four sick funds. The exact setting of this cap is a function of the budget decisions of the Ministry of Health. For a number of years, the HMOs have been realizing losses because they have run out of funds prior to the end of the year. However, under the new law, the government must fully reimburse the sick fund for any deficit incurred. In 1996, the combined sick fund deficit was more than $150 million, and the deficit for 1997 will be about $300 million [communication from Bruce Rosen].

As in Canada, health insurance in Israel is not employer based. Individuals join the HMO of their choice at annual open-enrollment periods. The premiums that individuals pay are on a sliding scale based on income. There are no deductibles or copayments for the basic benefit package. The Ministry of Health provides preventive health care services to Israeli citizens. Vaccines are provided free for contagious diseases such as measles and small pox. Maternity and children's preventive health care are provided by the government and are virtually free [Dov Chernichovsky and David Chinitz, "The Political Economy of Health System Reform in Israel," *Health Economics*, 4 (1995): 127–141, p. 128].

Israeli Health Care System: Summary

The Israeli health care system has the basic framework of a competitive managed health care system, but it often deviates from what the optimum amount of competition might be. Hospital rates are set by the government, which eliminates competitive selective contracting with hospitals by the sick funds. The absence of price competition among the sick funds reduces the incentives to contain costs in order to set lower prices to achieve a higher market share. There are, however, still some incentives to achieve lower costs in order to reap greater profits under the capped rate. The government, with little incentive for efficiency, still owns nearly one-half of all hospital beds.

Employers do not play a role in the health care system of Israel, and individuals can choose freely among the four plans at annual open-enrollment periods. Copayments are not used as a cost-containment device, but this appears to be society's choice. Preventive vaccinations for everyone are supplied by the Ministry of Health. The Israeli health care system appears to be much more equitable, since everyone is entitled to health care coverage and a limited risk adjustment measure is in place, but more inefficient than that of the United States. The managed competition system in Israel shows another country's divergence between the theoretical version of managed competition and the practical difficulties of actual implementation.

Dutch Health Care System

The Dutch health care system is an advanced model of a system that combines economic efficiency with distributional equity. Countries that seek to achieve efficiency and distributional equity may gain insight from the Dutch system, although the lessons that may be learned are far from complete.

Former Dutch Health Care System

The highly regulated former Dutch system included a compulsory sickness fund component with a standard benefit package of physician, hospital, prescription drugs, physiotherapy, and some dental services for employees (and their dependents) earning less than $30,000 a year (including those who were unemployed), in which 62 percent of the country was enrolled. A second program was the noncompulsory commercial insurance system with a flexible benefit package for self-employed individuals and higher-income groups, in which 32 percent of the population was enrolled with 50 insurers. Premiums could vary and insurers were free to avoid high-risk individuals. An additional 6 percent of the Dutch population (civil servants and their families) also had basic private insurance as compulsory insurance [Netherlands Ministry of Welfare, Health, and Cultural Affairs, *Changing Health Care in the Netherlands* (The Hague, The Netherlands: Ministry of Welfare, Health, and Cultural Affairs, 1988); W. P. M. M. van de Ven, "From Regulated Cartel to Regulated Competition in the Dutch Health Care System," *European Economic Review*, 34 (1990): 632–645]. In general, one-half of the premium of the sickness funds and the commercial health insurers was paid by the employer and one-half was paid by the employee. Sickness fund revenues were collected in a general fund, while premiums were paid directly to the insuring organizations themselves. In addition, the national health care program for all Dutch citizens, the Compulsory Exceptional Medical Expenses (Compensation) Act, covered nursing home care, special institutional care for disabled individuals, and prolonged hospital stays. It was financed by income-related premiums paid by employees. Fewer than 1 percent of Dutch citizens did not have health insurance.

The Dutch health care system generated a number of inefficiencies, yet still did not solve the problem of an inequitable distribution of health services. Regulation created barriers to competition from new potential entrants, existing providers, and managed care plans. Regulation also eliminated price competition among providers and choice of sickness funds by consumers. The sickness funds were each assigned a population from a particular region and by law were not allowed to compete against one another. The sickness funds had no incentive to be efficient. They were reimbursed by the capital general fund according to the health expenditures of their members. If sickness funds reduced costs through efficiency, reimbursement was reduced.

Sickness funds generally did not compete on a cost-containment basis. The uniform fees of physicians set by the government, the prohibition of limited provider plans, the potential boycott (due to the absence of antitrust legislation against providers) by providers against insurers if cost-containment activities were put into place, all inhibited cost containment. Commercial insurers competed in attracting low-risk individuals by age-related premiums and inserting preexisting condition clauses in their contracts. Healthy individuals who were eligible for private health insurance paid lower premiums than did lower-income individuals [B. L. Kirkman-Liff and W. P. M. M. van de Ven, "Improving Efficiency in the Dutch Health Care System: Current Innovations and Future Options," *Health Policy*, 13 (1989): 35–53; R. M. Lapre, "A Change in Direction in the Dutch Health care System?" *Health Policy*, 10 (1988): 21–32; Netherlands Ministry of Welfare, Health, and Cultural Affairs, *Changing Health Care in the Netherlands*; of W. P. M. M. van de Ven, "The Key Role of Health Insurance in a Cost-Effective Health Care System," *Health Policy*, 7 (1987): 253–272; W. P. M. M. van de Ven, "From Regulated Cartel to Regulated Competition in the Dutch Health Care System"].

Movement for Change in the Dutch Health Care System

In 1988, the Dutch government proposed an overhaul of their health care system for a number of reasons. First, health care costs had shown a sharp upward trend to more than 8 percent of the gross national product in the mid-1980s, one of the highest percentages among European countries. Second, the increased risk rating of premiums by commercial insurers created unacceptable inequities among the population. Third, the lack of incentives for cost containment by the sickness funds and the prohibitions against the limited provider plans made it difficult to contain costs. Fourth, the regulation of the supply of physicians and hospitals to contain costs became unworkable, insofar as the optimal number of providers was difficult to calculate. Moreover, the providers themselves found regulation to be onerous, and they became more amenable to a competitive alternative [Netherlands Ministry of Welfare, Health, and Cultural Affairs, *Changing Health Care in the Netherlands*; B. L. Kirkman-Liff and W. P. M. M. van de Ven, "Improving Efficiency in the Dutch Health Care System: Current Innovations and Future Options"; W. P. M. M. van de Ven, "The Dutch Health Care System," paper presented at George Washington University, Washington, DC, May 1991].

The health care system proposed by the Dutch government, would place greater stress on distributional equity, allocative efficiency, and competition among all insuring organizations (to be called "care insurers"). The new system is based on the consumer-choice health plan first proposed by Alain Enthoven ["Consumer Choice Health Plan," *New England Journal of Medicine*, 298 (1978): 650–658, 709–720]. Each individual or family would select a health plan from competing care insurers—HMOs, PPOs, or any form of indemnity plan—during an open-enrollment period every year. Distinctions in purchasing a health plan among those who are employed with a firm, self-employed, or unemployed would be eliminated. However, employers would be able to pay up to one-half of the health care premium for an employee if they desire. The government would require care insurers to offer a substantially similar benefit package to all Dutch citizens to prevent the practice of offering skimpy benefit packages to attract the healthiest persons. The benefit package would cover nearly all acute care, long-term care, and health care-related social welfare expenses. Individuals would also be free to purchase a supplemental plan that would cover discretionary cosmetic surgery, alternative medicine, and hospital amenities such as private rooms from among competing care insurers.

Individuals would pay an income-based premium into a central fund. They would also pay to the health plan of their choice a fee equal to approximately 10 percent of the average per capita costs of the covered benefits. This additional fee would be independent of income and could vary by care insurer, creating incentives for care insurers to be efficient in order to reduce their premiums. The additional fee could not be based on an individual's health status.

In the new health care system everyone would be entitled to health care coverage. Individuals with low incomes or are unemployed would pay only a modest premium into the central fund, although insurance would be compulsory to avoid the free-rider problem of receiving coverage without payment. Plans would be reimbursed by the central fund equal to the number of their enrollees adjusted by their case mix. In addition, the government would have the option to set a maximum to the additional fees, in effect a budget cap on each care insurer, equal to the degree of cost containment the government desired. The central fund reimbursement, therefore, would accomplish two goals. First, plans would have less incentive to avoid high-risk individuals, since capitation payment would be based in part on case mix. Second, plans would have incentives to contain costs. Moreover, plans that delivered services more efficiently and with higher quality would enroll a larger number of people.

Competing care insurers would be expected to enter into contracts with hospitals and physicians for efficiency-improving measures such as preadmission review and other forms of utilization management. Unlike the current system, the proposed system would allow care insurers to contract selectively with efficient providers. First, cost containment would be achieved by competition among capitated care insurers and by potential government limits on the use of the most expensive technology. Care insurers would not be allowed to deny coverage during the open-enrollment period, and insurers enrolling a disproportionate number of high-risk individuals would be compensated by the central fund according to case mix. If the case mix were calculated correctly, care insurers would have little incentive to avoid high-risk individuals.

Calculation of a case-mix adjustment is complex, however. Prior utilization of health services, functional health status (the ability to perform activities of daily living or the degree of one's infirmity), prior medical expenditure, disability, diagnostic information, and indicators of chronic medical conditions appear to be the most important factors in calculating the case-mix adjustment [W. P. M. M. van de Ven and R. C. J. A. van Vliet, "How Can We Prevent Cream Skimming in a Competitive Health Insurance Market?" paper presented at the Second World Congress on Health Economics, Zurich, September 1990]. Thus far, researchers have been able to explain approximately two-thirds of the maximum predictable variance of about 15 to 20 percent in individual health expenditures with case-mix measures. Approximately 85 percent of the variance in individual health care expenditures is simply unpredictable [J. P. Newhouse, W. G. Manning, E. B. Keeler, and E. M. Sloss, "Adjusting Capitation Rates Using Objective Health Resources and Prior Utilization," *Health Care Financing Review*, 10 (1989): 41–54; W. P. M. M. van de Ven and R. C. J. A. van Vliet, "How Can

We Prevent Cream Skimming in a Competitive Health Insurance Market?"] Case-mix measures, however, do not need to be perfect because care insurers also cannot forecast the case mix of their population and their future expenses with precision. Additional research on case-mix measurement is, however, clearly needed.

Under the proposed system, the Dutch government would act as the "sponsor" envisioned by Enthoven ["Managed Competition of Alternative Delivery Systems," in *Competition in the Health Care Sector: Ten Years Later*, ed. W. Greenberg (Durham, NC: Duke University Press, 1988), pp. 83–89]. It would ensure that the plans were financially viable, help individuals interpret the plans' provisions, determine the amount that the government and individuals would contribute, set the percentage sliding scale of premiums that individuals would pay, help individuals evaluate the quality of providers within each of the plans, and specify the basic benefit package of the health plans.

Care insurers would be expected to advertise the quality of their plans as well as the relative quality of health care providers with which they contract. New advances in technology that would be used by the care insurers would also be advertised to gain more business. Care insurers would emphasize convenience of location, short waiting times, and other amenities associated with the plan. Some care insurers may inform consumers about the efficacy of their cost-containment methods. In addition, a number of independent consulting firms may begin to provide advice to consumers on the relative advantages and disadvantages of the various care insurers. The government may evaluate care insurers and provide consumer protection to ensure that the insurers do not provide false and misleading advertising. The government would have an extensive antitrust role, especially in regard to anticompetitive hospital mergers and potential physician boycotts of cost-containment activities. The government would also have to monitor signs of potential collusion among care insurers.

The proposed Dutch health care system appears to have a number of advantages. It would preserve incentives for care insurers to compete on innovative cost-containment measures. Plans that are more successful in controlling costs can realize greater revenues as well as increased market shares. Plans could also compete on quality of providers, quality of service, convenience, or any other basis. At the same time, the system would attempt to eliminate competition among care insurers in avoiding high-risk individuals. There is a significant equity component in the proposed Dutch system since individuals would pay premiums based, in large part, on income. Individuals could not be refused health care insurance, and all individuals would have to purchase the standardized benefit package.

It is important to understand a number of other benefits of the new Dutch system. First, there would be no Medicare or Medicaid components and no DRG price controls or physician fee schedules that create incentives to shift costs to other areas of the health care sector. There would be incentives to use resources in their most efficient setting. Depending on how high or low it is set, a budget cap could force the health plans to eliminate services for which there are some marginal benefits but for which costs to society substantially exceed the benefits. This would mean that every care insurer would have to ration or limit care within the organization. With a cap on both acute and long-term care expenditures, the organization itself would decide how best to allocate resources to maximize its income or number of enrollees or to achieve other goals.

Importance of Risk Adjustment in Care Insurer Competition

The Dutch health care system addresses the potential for cream skimming by the sick funds in a number of ways. First, the twenty-five sick funds must have homogeneous benefits packages. This prevents altering the benefits package (such as offering dental benefits for younger children) in order to attract younger families. Benefits are stated in terms of types of services received rather than by the type of medical practitioner who provides the services in order to give firms flexibility in substituting medical inputs. Homogeneity of benefits, however, eliminates consumer choice among types of basic benefits plans.

Second, it is against the law to deny health insurance coverage to individuals regardless of health status. Moreover, there is an open-enrollment period every year to guard against adverse selection when individuals choose plans. Individuals cannot immediately quit one plan and join another when first hearing about an illness.

Sick funds still find subtle ways to avoid high-risk individuals. They may be rude to sicker individuals; they may keep more sickly individuals waiting before authorizing specialist treatment; they may contract with suboptimal providers. Locating treatment facilities in neighborhoods with younger families may help attract a favorable case mix. Thus, beginning in 1993, the Netherlands instituted a risk adjustment measure for competing sick funds. Monies are distributed from the central fund to each of the sick funds based on age, gender, geographic location, and disability indicators of their enrollees, which still, however, does not account for all of the case-mix variance. With an improved risk adjustment measure, managed care firms have greater incentives to improve their quality of care. Sick funds no longer have incentives to produce a lower quality of care because less healthy enrollees provide a greater risk-adjustment reimbursement. They also have greater incentives to advertise and provide information on the higher quality of care that is produced. Firms may seek to develop a reputation in managed care quality. One would therefore expect a number of sick funds to produce higher quality of care at somewhat higher prices and others to produce lower quality of care at somewhat lower prices.

Lessons of the Dutch Health Care System for the U.S. System

The Dutch health care system points up two large deficiencies in the U.S. health care system. The first is reliance on employer-based as opposed to individual-based coverage. The Dutch health care system relies on individual-based coverage and shows that there are no good economic reasons for retaining the employer-based system and its attendant costs in the United States. Lost productivity and other inefficiencies, including imperfections in the tax system, are not part of an individual-based system. Second, the Dutch system uses a risk-adjusted measure to prevent cream skimming. Although difficult to implement in practice, risk adjustment may lead to greater coverage of those who are uninsured and improved quality and information in the health care marketplace.

Summary

The health care systems of Canada, Israel, and the Netherlands are three alternatives to the U.S. health care system. Canada utilizes a single-payer system; in Israel, four managed care firms compete on a nonprice basis; in the Netherlands, sick funds compete on a price and nonprice basis. Because of the long-established single-payer system in Canada and the relatively mild forms of managed care cost containment in Israel and the Netherlands, there have been fewer hospital mergers or integrated physician-hospital organizations than in the United States. Each of the three countries struggles to achieve what they consider to be an optimal amount of government intervention, efficiency, and equity. Efficiency and equity are valued differently in each country. Unlike the United States, Canada, Israel, and the Netherlands place greater stress on a more equal distribution of health care services than on an efficient allocation of health care services.

Although the health care marketplace has changed considerably in the United States over the last decade, the microeconomic analysis has remained the same. The health care industry still must respond to the goals of physicians, profit-maximizing and nonprofit firms, utility-maximizing patients, technological advances, and movements and shifts in the demand for and supply of health care services. The industrial organization of the health care industry, complicated by the phenomenon of health insurance, is as complex as any other industry in the economy. Moreover, the greater concern in this industry over the "correct" distribution of services separates the analysis of the health care industry from many others.

Index

A

Adjusted average per capita cost (AAPCC), 80–81
AFDC (Aid to Families with Dependent Children) benefits, 73
AHCCCS (Arizona Health Care Cost Containment System), 83–84
Aid to Families with Dependent Children (AFDC) benefits, 73
AMA, *see* American Medical Association
American Medical Association (AMA), 21
   in regard to alleged violation of Federal Trade Commission Act, 22–26
Anderson, Gerard F., 124
Antitrust, vii
   demand and, 105–107
   evaluation of, 115–116
   in health care sector, 103–117
   legal and economic impediments to, 104–105
   perspective on vertical integration, 114–115
   supply and, 107–114
Arizona Health Care Cost Containment System (AHCCCS), 83–84
Arrow, Kenneth J., 4, 132
Average net income, 18

B

Baker, Lawrence C., 55
Barriers to entry to industry, 5
Berg, Stacy, 86
Berk, Marc L., 51, 148
Bishop, Christine E., 91
Blue Cross and Blue Shield, 44–45

Blue Cross & Blue Shield United of Wisconsin v. *Marshfield Clinic* and *Security Health Plan of Wisconsin, Inc.*, 116–117, 118
Blue Cross of Maryland, Inc., et al., v. *Franklin Square Hospital et al.*, 132, 133–134
Blumstein, James F., 145
Bodenheimer, Thomas, 58
Boren Amendment, 86
Buchanan, Joan L., 83
Buchmueller, Thomas C., 56
Burge, Russel T., 13

C

Canadian health care system, 152, 153–154, 164
CCRCs (continuing care retirement communities), 98–99
Clayton Act, 103
Clinton health care reform plan, 130–131
CMPs (competitive medical plans), 46
Cohen, J. W., 84
Collusion, 8
Competition in health care sector, 127–129
Competitive medical plans (CMPs), 46
Consolidated Omnibus Budget Reconciliation Act (COBRA), 66
Continuing care retirement communities (CCRCs), 98–99
Cooper, Philip F., 65
Corts, Kenneth S., 55
Cost-conscious behavior, Medicare program and, 76–79
Cost-conscious managed care, viii

166 Index

Cream skimming
  managed care and, 51–52
  potential antidotes to, 52–54
Creative destruction, process of, 10
Cromwell, Jerry, 15
Cross-elasticity
  of demand, 30–31
  of supply, 31
Cutler, David M., 44, 69, 137

D

Davis, Karen, 58
Demand
  antitrust and, 105–107
  cross-elasticity of, 30–31
  elasticity of, 3
  facing long-term care industry, 96
  rationing and, 144–149
  supplier-induced, 14–15
Demand curve, 2–3
  shift in, 4
Diagnosis-related group (DRG) system of payment, 77–78, 82
Diamond, Peter, 65
Dowd, Bryan, 54–55, 56
Dranove, David, 34
DRG (diagnosis-related group) system of payment, 77–78, 82
Dutch health care system, 152, 158–164

E

Economic impediments to antitrust, 104–105
Economics of health care, 1–11
Economist's view of health care marketplace, vii–viii
Elasticity of demand and supply, 3
Ellis, Randall P., 48
Employee Retirement Income Security Act (ERISA), 48, 144
Employer-based health insurance, 63–69
Employer-based long-term care insurance, 95–96
Enthoven, Alain C., 128
Enthoven's consumer choice health plan, 129–130
Equilibrium price, 4

Expenditures
  health care, 1, 2
  in long-term care industry, 91
Externalities, 9

F

Feder, Judith, 58
Federal Employees Health Benefits Program (FEHBP), 68
Federal Trade Commission Act, 103–104
Feldman, Roger, 54–55, 56
Feldstein, Martin S., 64
Feldstein, Paul J., 56
Fisher, C. R., 148
Flexner Report, 122
Frank, Richard G., 28
Friedlob, A., 99
Fuchs, Victor R., 57, 146

G

Garnick, Deborah W., 21
GDP (gross domestic product), 1, 2
Gonzales, Theresa I., 81
Government regulation, *see* Regulation
Greenberg, Warren, viii
Gross domestic product (GDP), 1, 2
Group practice, 13
Gruber, Jonathan, 69

H

Hadley, Jack, 58, 125
Harrington, C., 99
Harris, Jeffrey, 27
Health care
  competition in, 127–129
  distribution of, 9–10
  economics of, 1–11
  employer and employee as purchasers of, 63–70
  industrial organization of, 1
  nonprice rationing in, 145–149
  regulation in, 122–126
  size and growth of, 1, 2
  technology and rationing in, 135–149
Health care costs
  rising, technology and, 135–137
  trends in, 140–144
Health care expenditures, 1, 2

Health care marketplace
  Canadian, 152, 153–154, 164
  demand and supply in, 2–9
  Dutch, 152, 158–164
  economist's view of, vii–viii
  Israeli, 152, 155–158, 164
Health care reform, viii
Health insurance, 5, viii
  employer-based, 63–69
  in health care sector, 43–48
  in public sector, 73–88
  uninsured and, 57–59
Health Insurance Portability and Accountability Act, 66
Health maintenance organizations (HMOs), 10, 13, 46–47, 49
  choice of insuring organization and, 56
  Medicare, 79–81
Health Security Act, 130–131
Held, P. J., 146
Hellinger, Fred J., 19, 52
Hiatt, Howard H., 20
High-risk pooling, mandatory, 53–54
Hillman, Alan L., 47, 137
Hirschman Herfindahl Index (HHI), 85
HMOs, see Health maintenance organizations
Holahan, J. F., 84
Home health care, Medicare program and, 81
Hospital industry, 27–35
  changes in structure of, 28–30
  characteristics of, 27–28
Hospitals
  competition among, 30–34
  recent performance of, 34–35
  regulation of, 86–87
Hughes, Edward F. X., 125

I
Income, average net, 18
Industrial organization of health care, 1
Industry, barriers to entry to, 5
Information, vii
  asymmetry of, 14
Insurance
  health, see Health insurance
  long-term care, see Long-term care insurance

Insurance regulation, 126–127
Israeli health care system, 152, 155–158, 164

J
Job lock phenomenon, 65–66
  reverse, 66
Joint Committee on Accreditation of Healthcare Organizations (JCAHO), 32–33

K
Kassenbaum-Kennedy Bill, 66, 96
Kemper, Peter, 92
Kennedy, R. H., 33
Kessel, Reuben A., 7
Kronick, Richard, 64, 128

L
Legal impediments to antitrust, 104–105
Legal intervention, vii
Life Care at Home model, 99
Long-term care industry, 91–100
  alternatives in, 98–99
  demand facing, 96
  economic attributes of, 92–94
  expenditures in, 91
  future of, 99–100
  supply in, 97
Long-term care insurance, 93, 94–96
  employer-based, 95–96
  private, 95
Luft, Harold S., 49, 55

M
Malpractice, physicians and, 20–21
Managed care, 45–48
  competition and, 48–49
  competition effects of, 54–56
  cost-conscious, viii
  cream skimming and, 51–52
  health care marketplace and, 10–11
Manning, Willard G., 44, 48
Market incentives, physicians and, 19
Massachusetts v. *Dukakis*, 88, 89–90
McBride, Timothy D., 58
McCarran-Ferguson Act, 105
McClennan, Mark, 136
McGann v. *H&H Music Company, et al.*, 67, 70, 71–72

McGuire, Thomas G., 48
Medi-Cal program, 84
Medicaid program, 16–17, 58, 82–86, 94–95, 99
   expenditures, 86
Medical technology, *see* Technology
Medicare program, 17, 58, 73, 74–82, 95
   competitive approach and, 79–81
   cost-conscious behavior and, 76–79
   financing of, 75–76
   home health care and, 81
   summary of state of, 81–82
Medicare reimbursement, technology and, 138–139
Medicare volume performance standards (MVPS), 17–18, 78
Mendelson, Daniel N., 142
Mennemeyer, Stephen T., 84
Mergers, 29
Meyer, Jack A., 70*n*
Miller, Robert H., 49
Mitchell, Janet B., 15, 83
Mitchell, Jean M., 15
Monheit, Alan C., 51, 65
x Monopolistic competition model, 8
Monopoly model, 6–7
Monopsony pricing, 50–51
Moral hazard, 43
Morrisey, Michael A., 34
Murtaugh, Christopher M., 92
MVPS (Medicare volume performance standards), 17–18, 78

N
National Practitioner Data Bank, 20
Net income, average, 18
Netanyahu Commission, 156
Netherlands health care system, 152, 158–164
Newcomer, R., 99
Newhouse, Joseph P., 20, 53, 141
Nonhospital providers, supply of, 112–113
Nonphysician providers, supply of, 110
Nonprice rationing in health care, 145–149
Nursing homes, *see* Long-term care industry

O
Ocean State Physicians Health Plan, Inc., et al. v. Blue Cross and Blue Shield of Rhode Island, 59–60, 61–62
Oligopoly model, 8–9

P
Patients, physicians as agents for, 15–16
Pauly, Mark V., 4, 5, 15, 45, 47
Peltzman, Sam, 121
Perrin, J. M., 138
Pharmaceutical industry, technology and, 139–140
Phibbs, Ciaran, 84–85
PHOs, *see*Physician-hospital organizations
Physician-hospital organizations (PHOs), 13–14
   supply of, 113
Physician services industry, 12–21
   structure of, 12–14
Physicians
   as agents for patients, 15–16
   competition among, 19–20
   malpractice and, 20–21
   market incentives and, 19
   paying, 16–18
   supply of, 110–112
Point-of-service plans (POS), 47
Pope, Gregory C., 13
Porell, Irame W., 80
POS (point-of-service plans), 47
Preferred provider organizations (PPOs), 13, 47, 84
Price
   equilibrium, 4
   regulation of, 123–125
Pricing, monopsony, 50–51
Public goods, 9
Public health insurance programs, 73–88
Pure competition model, 5–6

R
Rationing, demand and, 144–149
RBRVS (resource-based relative value scale), 17, 18, 78, 124
Reform, health care, viii

Regulation
    in health care sector, 122–126
    of industries other than health care, 119–121
    insurance, 126–127
    of price, 123–125
    restricting entry into provider markets, 122–123
Reinhardt, Uwe E., 131
Resource-based relative value scale (RBRVS), 17, 18, 78, 124
Risk adjustment measure, 53
Rivlin, A. M., 98
Robinson, James C., 55–56, 84–85
Russell, L. B., 137

S
S/HMOs (social/health maintenance organizations), 98–99
Salkever, David S., 28
Scanlon, William J., 91
Schneiderman, Lawrence J., 148
Schorr, Alvin L., 64
Schumpeter, Joseph, 10
Schwartz, J. S., 137
Schwartz, William B., 142
Scott, Elton, 15
Self-insured plans, 48
Shayne, May W., 94
Sherman Act, 103
Shortell, Stephen, 125
Sloan, Frank A., 20, 94, 98, 125, 138, 145
Social benefits, 9
Social/health maintenance organizations (S/HMOs), 98–99
Spenddown, 94
Steinberg, Earl, 58
Supplier-induced demand, 14–15
Supply
    antitrust and, 107–114
    cross-elasticity of, 31
    elasticity of, 3
    in long-term care industry, 97
    of nonhospital providers, 112–113
    of nonphysician providers, 110
    of physicians, 110–112

Supply curve, 2–3
    shift in, 4
Swartz, Katherine, 58, 125
System integration, 56–57

T
Technology, 136
    diffusion of, 137–138
    Medicare reimbursement and, 138–139
    pharmaceutical industry and, 139–140
    rising health care costs and, 135–137
TennCare program, 85–86
Tompkins, Christopher P., 80

U
UCR (usual, customary, and reasonable) basis, 16
U.S. and State of Connecticut v. HealthCare Partners, Inc. Danbury Area IPA, Inc., and Danbury Health Systems, Inc., 114
U.S. v. Carilion Health System, 29, 35, 36–38
U.S. v. Health Choice of Northwest Missouri, Inc., Heartland Health System, Inc., and St. Joseph Physicians, Inc., 113–114
U.S. v. Montana Nursing Home Association, 100, 101–102
U.S. v. Rockford Memorial Corp., 29, 35, 39–42
Usual, customary, and reasonable (UCR) basis, 16

V
Valvona, J., 138
Veterans Administration (VA), 73
Vita, Michael G., 125
Vogel, Ronald J., 97

W
Wade, Marcia, 86
Weisbrod, Burton A., 136
Welch, W. Pete, 47
Weller, Paul C., 20

White, William D., 34
Wholey, Douglas, 55
Wickizer, Thomas M., 49
Wickline v. *California*, 143–144, 149, 150–151
Wiener, J. M., 98

Williamson, Oliver E., 30
Wu, Lawrence, 34

Z

Zuckerman, Stephen, 86–87
Zwanziger, Jack, 85

10/7/98

indemnity = (n.) security from damage or loss : compensation for loss or injury : legal exemption from incurred liabilities or penalties

positive economics : knowledge
normative economics : analysis, judgments
NB economy of scale :